Celiac Creations For Multiple Food Allergies

How To Survive When Your Food Is Killing You

Gluten Free

Sugar Free

Chemical Sweetener Free

Dairy Free

Soy Free

Peanut Free

Tree Nut Free

Alcohol Free

by

June Ramey and Kristine Dzagan

Celiac Creations
For Multiple Food Allergies:
How to Survive When Your Food is Killing You

ISBN 978-1622-875-19-1 PRINT
ISBN 978-1622-875-20-7 EBOOK

LCCN 2014947325

March 2015

Published and Distributed by
First Edition Design Publishing, Inc.
P.O. Box 20217, Sarasota, FL 34276-3217
www.firsteditiondesignpublishing.com

This book is not intended as a substitute for the medical advice of physicians. The reader should regularly consult a physician in matters relating to his/her health and particularly with respect to any symptoms that may require diagnosis or medical attention.

We dedicate this book to:

Father who protected us through our journey and continues to watch over us

Mashiach Yeshua (Jesus Christ) who carried us through the tough times

Ruach Ha Kodesh (The Holy Spirit) who provided us with inspiration in the kitchen

and

Bob who was the love of my life and who, with Adonai's help,
taught me the true meaning of love.

FOREWORD

It is my pleasure to write a Foreword for this cookbook. I have known Kris for some time and watched her as she struggled with complex and challenging food allergies. She and her mother, June, have worked diligently to find recipes and food combinations that allow for diversity and varied tastes without incorporating her food allergens.

Food allergies can be debilitating for many and often go undiagnosed. Common food allergy symptoms include gas, abdominal bloating, constipation, diarrhea, skin rashes (like eczema), joint pain, chronic sinus infections, and headaches. Food allergies are associated with inflammation and, if undiagnosed and eaten over a lifetime, can increase one's risk of more chronic health scenarios like asthma, irritable bowel syndrome, rheumatoid arthritis, and cancer.

Foods that are eliminated in this book include gluten, sugar, dairy, soy, peanuts, alcohol, and sorghum, with recipes made mostly from scratch. With all of these challenges addressed—even if you do not have food allergies—you will find the recipes extremely delicious. As Kris and June have recommended, adjust recipes to your needs as they themselves have done. If you are vegetarian, replace beef broth with vegetable stock and replace beef with tempeh or TVP (texturized vegetable protein, both soy products). If you are diabetic, avoid the bread and pasta recipes. If you have an egg allergy, replace each egg (in baked items) with 1 tablespoon flax meal soaked in 3 tablespoons hot water. Personally, I choose not to eat meat, so I replaced the bacon in the Creamy Lentil Soup recipe with flavored tempeh, and it was wonderful. Be playful and enjoy your time in the kitchen.

As a Naturopathic Doctor, I believe food is one of the foundations of optimal health. Food allergies were considered unimportant and not addressed for a long time in our conventional medical system. It is very apparent now that these are real issues and Celiac Disease is one of the most dangerous, for it triggers an immune reaction that attacks the small intestine. If you feel you have food allergies, it is highly recommended that you discuss this with your Naturopathic or Medical doctor. It is important to choose a doctor who understands current research and is willing to run appropriate blood tests in order to look for the various forms of allergies.

I am so thankful to Kris and June for taking the time and energy to put their recipes on paper. Their hard work shows in the delicious options they offer throughout this cookbook. For anyone who has recently been diagnosed with Celiac Disease or other food allergies, this is an excellent resource.

In Health,
Stephany Porter, ND, FABNO
Naturopathic Doctor

The Bodhi Clinic
Millersville, Maryland
www.bodhiclinic.com

About the Authors

June Ramey is a great-grandmother with a long history of creative cooking. At age 4 she discovered combining mud with Crisco was not a good idea. By age 13, she was cooking for real using fresh herbs out of the garden. As a 19-year vegetarian, she has learned to balance proteins and carbs. Always loving a challenge, she has successfully taken on the world of creative gluten-free cooking with extensive food allergies. Her love of cooking is evident in the recipes she's engineered.

Professionally, she's an executive administrative assistant and lives with her daughter, Kris, and her grandson, Jonathan, in Ellicott City, Maryland. In her words, "Life doesn't get any better than living with the people you love!"

Kris Dzagan grew up in farmlands of North Dakota and suburbs of small Minnesota towns most of her childhood but has fond memories of playing on her uncle's dairy farm with her cousins in the 1970s. That's where she began to enjoy the wholesome taste of fresh cooked farm foods. At about that same time, the family experimented with natural foods, although there were not nearly as many items on the market as there are today.

Kris joined the military when she was 17 years old and traveled to various places around the world, enjoying and tasting the cuisine of several European and Asian countries. After retiring from the military, she married Bob Dzagan and moved to Ellicott City, Maryland. Kris has three children and two grandchildren.

Kris was diagnosed with Celiac Disease in 2010. Since then, she has continued to discover additional food sensitivities and allergies that are not included in this cookbook. In the beginning of this gastronomic journey, she would have rather fixed the roof or worked in her well-equipped workshop than spend time in the kitchen. However, cooking with fresh and interesting ingredients has ignited a creative spark in her and created an environment for collaboration and testing, turning their kitchen into a classroom and lab. She continues to develop and experiment with new recipes.

ACKNOWLEDGEMENTS

Sincere thanks are in order to the following people:

Jonathan McLean, resident tester and co-designer of recipes and recipe names. Without his feedback, we would have never received the Kid's Stamp of Approval.

Mary Butzer, SSND, BA, M.ED, MAPS for her wisdom, knowledge, and encouragement in the writing process. I would have never expected to draw on her excellent education, but being a long time teacher, before I knew what had happened, she was gently teaching me and letting me think it was all my idea.

Julia Murray for her willingness to be our head taste tester and give us insightful feedback. Julia does not have dietary restrictions, and we knew if it passed the Julia Test the recipe was a keeper!

Barry Thornton, our very good family friend, who braved the uniqueness of our cooking with subtle humor. His help in the kitchen during meal preparation provided excellent feedback from a man's perspective.

Didon Pachner, who also doesn't have dietary restrictions but was willing to try something new. Her honest feedback made us think about our recipes from a different perspective.

Maureen Burke from One Dish Cuisine for her encouragement, taste testing, and willingness to engineer recipe fixes that had us perpetually stumped. Her generosity in sharing her vast knowledge and years of experience in the gluten-free world was invaluable to us.

Dr. John E. Humiston, founder of CandidaMD, for graciously allowing us to share his extensive knowledge about Candida, including its causes and effects. We very much appreciate what this forward-thinking physician is doing to educate the public and his fellow physicians.

INTRODUCTION

In 2014, Celiac Disease, Gluten Sensitivity, Food Allergies, and Autism are being diagnosed at epidemic levels. This is evident to me every day as I meet customers who come into my gluten and allergen-free Café, Deli, and Bakery, desperately looking for a safe and healthy meal to eat. I definitely understand because I have lived with Celiac Disease, several food allergies, and many food intolerances since the late 1980s. Some of my customers are just sick and tired of being sick and tired, and are finding relief on gluten and casein-free diets, etc. A cookbook covering more than a few allergies is long overdue.

It is very difficult managing a simple gluten-free diet (no wheat, rye, barley), but when you add in severe food allergies such as casein (dairy and milk), soy, eggs, peanuts, tree nuts, fish, and shellfish along with corn, sulfites, nitrates, oats, legumes, caffeine and meat protein, that's when the real challenge begins and when I have the most fun! However, I know it is not fun for those who are suddenly thrown into this way of cooking, and it can seem like there is nothing safe or healthy to eat. Unfortunately, we live in a world of overly processed food, and that processing often adds many unnecessary ingredients and allergens to preserve them or to make the product at a lower cost. Thus, it is virtually impossible for those with Celiac Disease and multiple food allergies to eat outside their homes and, sometimes, even within their own homes, leaving a huge challenge for parents/caregivers when it comes to safely feeding their loved one.

I have been a willing taste tester, and June and Kris have done a great job with this cookbook. You will find the recipes are very easy to follow. Keep in mind that if you cannot have eggs, you can use Egg Replacer Powder and water (double it for gluten-free baking), and sometimes you can just omit the egg in a lasagna or casserole and it is just fine. If you cannot have corn, you can use tapioca starch to replace cornstarch, and substitute baking soda and cream of tartar for baking powder. Once you master the recipes in this book, you have the basics you need to create your own meals at home.

I am honored to be a very small part of this book and am so thrilled that you will be able to benefit from June's and Kris's hard work. Once you try some of these recipes, you will have an “ah ha” moment and will be empowered to begin converting your own recipes with the substitutions you have learned.

As I say at the Café, “Relax and feel the difference and welcome back to the table.”

Maureen Burke
Chef/Owner
One Dish Cuisine Café, Deli & Bakery

Gluten Free, Allergen Free
Ellicott City, Maryland
www.onedishcuisinegfcfsf.com

How To Use This Cookbook

- Rule # 1: Have fun! Don't be afraid to experiment and make mistakes. Some of our best recipes were mistakes.
- Rule # 2: Don't be intimidated by the number of ingredients or steps in a recipe. We've designed the recipes and instructions to be user friendly, suitable for novice cooks and advanced chefs.
- Rule # 3: Write in your cookbook. We suggest the first time you make a recipe, make it as written. If you feel it needs improvement, write in the cookbook to adapt to your taste. The second time you make that dish, follow your adaptations.
- Rule # 4: Think outside the box. Many of the desserts and snacks are so healthy, they can be eaten for breakfast. (Who wouldn't want Sweet Potato Pie or Irresistible Granola for breakfast?)

How To Read The Recipe

- Ingredients are listed in the order in which they will be used.
- All ingredients for a particular step are grouped together.
- Some recipes will have a double column within a partitioned area. All ingredients should be used in that step.

How To Prepare To Cook

- Read the recipe in its entirety before beginning, as some recipes require use of additional recipes within the book. For example, many recipes list seasoned salt or a specific flour mixture. The recipe you're working with will reference the section where the recipe may be found.
- Set out all ingredients and kitchen tools before beginning the recipe. This will reduce the prep time.
- Ensure you have sufficient amounts of all mixtures, such as flour mixes, before you begin.
- We have made every effort to accurately describe prep time; however, if you are unfamiliar with some of the ingredients or a novice in the kitchen, allow yourself a bit more time.

- Washing, peeling and chopping fresh vegetables has been calculated in the prep time, but may take a little longer if you're not comfortable using kitchen tools.
- Become familiar with the "How To" section for helpful tips on how to prepare fresh parsley, care for wooden kitchen utensils, etc.

Using The Recipe To Cook

- Variations to the recipe and notes are listed at the end of the recipe.
- Use fresh herbs whenever you can. It will enhance the flavor of the meal.

Celiac Creations For Multiple Food Allergies

How To Survive When Your Food Is Killing You

June Ramey and Kristine Dzagan

Table of Contents

The Journey Begins

Life is an adventure. Each step brings us closer to unchartered territory: a place we've never been before. For some journeys, we walk through hardship and pain. Others inspire us with hope and purpose, but no matter what we're experiencing, attitude is everything. We have the freedom to choose what to think and how we will respond to our circumstances and to those around us. This cookbook began from two different walks of life that merged to overcome a seemingly impossible situation and to provide hope for others who may be traveling a similar path.

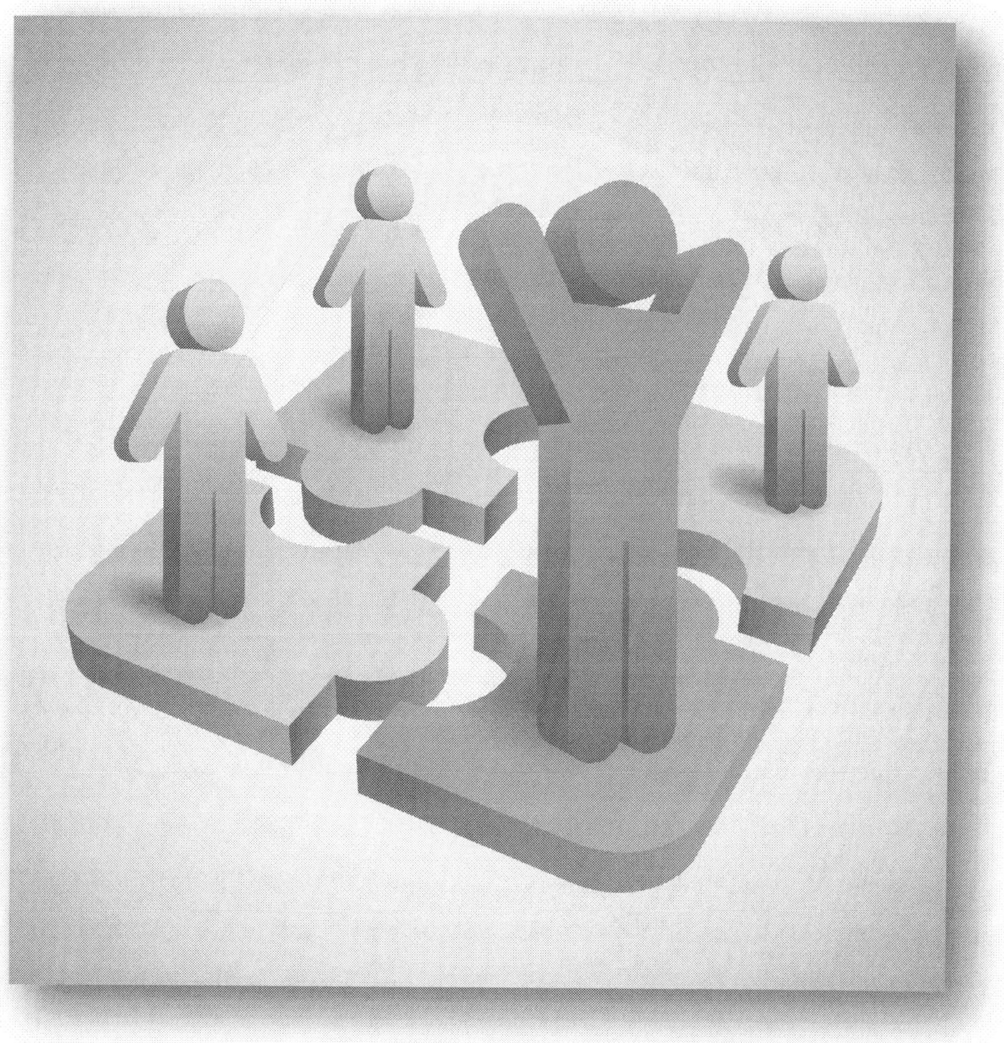

The Beginning of Kris's Journey

Isolation

"There's nothing to eat! I'm going to starve to death!" I honestly felt alone and overwhelmed, like I had just been shipwrecked on a deserted island. No food, no help, nowhere to turn. I was exhausted and continually ill as emotions welled up within me. I could almost feel the very ground on which I stood was shaking. My world was changing and there wasn't anything I could do about it. Every food I loved and craved was on my "do not eat" list. The sudden realization that things would never be the same again filled me with a sense of dread and helplessness. How does a person with multiple food allergies and restrictions move from a desperate situation of starvation to one of enjoyment and plenty? It involves a change of heart and mindset to have fun and explore this new world. It is possible to find joy in the journey!

The road from a dry, barren land to a lush garden of opportunity began several years earlier. When my husband and I married, he was incredibly active. In his early 50s, he was carrying 120 pound bags of sand on his shoulders to set pavers for a new patio and was able to hike 18 miles in the wilderness. It seemed he had boundless energy and strength. One summer evening, we were sitting outside enjoying the evening sunset. The warm air kissed us with a gentle breeze, making it the perfect evening. In the middle of our conversation, his face wrinkled with pain and I helped him into the house. His left leg went rigid with excruciating pain—another agonizing charlie horse! I rushed to my knees on the floor to force his rigid leg and foot muscles to relax until the charlie horse passed. This was occurring more and more often and we were just beginning to visit the doctors to find out what was wrong. When I looked up at him, he was slumped to the left, his left arm limp and he was slurring his words. "Oh Lord," I prayed. "Please don't let him die on me! We've only been married for six months!"

Much to my relief and joy, the Good Lord heard my prayer and my husband survived the heart attack. But little did I realize this was just the beginning of our character building.

Shortly after that, my husband's health took a sudden turn for the worse. Within a year and a half, he went from being physically fit to barely being able to walk up a flight of stairs. We visited doctor after doctor trying to identify the source of his multiple illnesses. He patiently and silently endured invasive and non-invasive procedures all in the hope of finding a solution to his increasing disability and chronic pain. The number of his prescription drugs, which included narcotics and other heavy-duty medications, increased as we visited more doctors. The doctors were well qualified and compassionate, but none could identify the source of his chronic pain and progressively debilitating state. All tests given him were maddeningly inconclusive. Even so, he received disability retirement both through his job and from Social Security.

As my husband's health continued to deteriorate, I was often concerned about leaving him when I went to work. It was not so much that he couldn't take care of himself, it was more that my heart ached when we were separated. We were both chronically fatigued. I struggled to work full-time, to take care of my husband and my six-year-old son, to pay the bills, and to maintain the house and yard. My husband and I agreed that I needed help around the house, so we asked my mother to move in with us. She kindly agreed and, not long after, began helping around the house, yard and taking care of my son. We were a close family, doing everything together. Our motto was, "Consider others before you consider yourself."

The First Step

There is nothing more painful than watching the love of your life slowly die before your eyes. I was determined to improve the quality of life for my soul mate, and it became obvious that pharmaceuticals alone were not the answer. I thought if my husband's health could improve through the foods he ate, perhaps he could stop taking some of the medications and start on the road to recovery. So I began researching different conditions, such as fibromyalgia and Candida, to see if I could pinpoint the source of some of his illnesses and to determine which foods contributed to the symptoms associated with his medical conditions. My husband believed in nutrition, so we supplemented our diet with good quality vitamins and probiotics. But this wasn't enough.

For our first experiment, we removed gluten from our diet. Some of my true love's symptoms started to improve! There was a reduction in his seasonal allergy responses, such as chronic sinus drainage and coughing. What a relief! We were on the right path! This small victory echoed within me—my health conditions also improved! My Irritable Bowel Syndrome (IBS) symptoms were improving!

As joyful as we were with this discovery, our efforts were too little, too late, and the victory was short lived. Within two months, my husband's condition quickly declined. He was rushed to the emergency room and died two weeks later in the Intensive Care Unit from a fatal case of pancreatitis and septic shock.

With grief heavy on me like a burial shroud, I had no appetite and no motivation. My son was also experiencing intense grief and we both had little desire for anything, including food.

My sweet mother, still living with us, spent many hours in the kitchen cooking for us to make sure we didn't starve. This was a blessing for me. We are incredibly fortunate that she has always loved a cooking challenge and tackles every problem head-on.

Another Turn in the Road

We had just embraced a gluten-free diet at home when my husband passed away, and since I felt better eating gluten-free, we continued down this uncharted path. It was shortly thereafter that I discovered I had a soy intolerance, so we removed all soy from our diets. Although we cooked gluten and soy free at home, my mother and son had unrestricted diets. After ten months of being gluten free, I was officially diagnosed with Celiac Disease.

Although my health improved from eliminating gluten and soy, I still wasn't feeling well. I researched common food allergies and chose one food to target. I eliminated the food for a week or more, reintroduced the food into my diet, observed my body's responses and then decided if it was a "safe" food. This process took months and months of experimentation. Additional medical tests confirmed more allergies. As we continued to test my allergies to different foods, my list of safe foods dwindled down to mostly animal proteins, seeds, and most vegetables. At the time of this printing, my food allergies, intolerances, and sensitivities include gluten, dairy, soy, peanuts, tree nuts, cane sugar, artificial sweeteners (xylitol, sucralose, Splenda, etc), green tea, some seasonings (ginger, ginseng and thyme) tomatoes, mushrooms, most fruit, anything fermented (vinegar, alcohol, etc), yeast, and most corn products. As you can imagine, we had to become very creative in finding foods I could eat, which necessitated redesigning almost every recipe we used.

Parallel Paths

During the early stages of my food experiments, for about one and a half years, I had to take two or three days off work every month. My son would get a mysterious illness in which his temperature would suddenly spike to 103 or 104. His nose would run and he would throw up, or he would get white spots at the back of his throat. We'd take him to the doctor only to be told that it was probably a virus that had to run its course because the bacterial tests came back negative. We began documenting and tracking his symptoms, and, by the time we were able to predict when he would become ill again, we had a plan.

On a whim, and holding our breath, we decided to remove all gluten from his diet. Several weeks passed and I found I didn't have to take leave. Several more weeks passed and still he went to school every day. After three months, we concluded my son was gluten intolerant since he had not been formally diagnosed as Celiac.

Once we recognized that my son had food sensitivities, it was a small leap to discover that most soy products, with the exception of soy lecithin, also made him incredibly ill. The symptoms were slightly different, with intense abdominal pain under the left rib cage and diarrhea. He would often stay home from school for a couple of days after he had ingested soy. It was at that point we decided his lips should never touch gluten or soy products again.

From Desperation and Starvation to Experimentation, Adventure, and Success!

Each of us has our own unique story to tell, our journey through the deserts, mountains of hardship and the unexpected moments of hope and inspiration rest on us like early morning dew. We share a common bond—the insatiable drive for survival and the compelling hope that we can improve our situation. The sum of our lives is not encapsulated in this moment in time when we feel the most helpless and where our restrictions seem more like a prison sentence than a new beginning. So, how do we transition from victim to victor?

Embrace the challenge! Think about it. If life was always the same, never changing, it would be boring. (How many days in a row can you eat your favorite food?) This is a new adventure and opportunity for you to learn something exciting, to explore the unknown. It doesn't have to be scary or dreadful. Find a way to make it fun.

When we first started down this road and I realized I couldn't eat anything with gluten in it, I hated cooking. In fact, I would have rather done yard work and fixed the roof than spend an hour in the kitchen chopping vegetables and making dinner. I knew how to make about five meals and most of them were prepackaged or very simple. I had lost my enthusiasm for eating, except for foods that were high in carbohydrates and sugars. I lived for that "instant gratification" and "sugar rush."

Once I realized I either had to start cooking differently or starve, I accepted the challenge. In fact, I was determined that this setback wasn't going to beat me! We started cooking from scratch, reading every ingredient on every label, and coming up with creative new ways to fix an old meal.

Make it fun! It became a family game for every member to rate the meal on a scale of one to ten, with one meaning you were going to throw up and ten meaning you would pay a lot of money for that meal in a fancy restaurant. Anything that rated six and under was either thrown in the "do not make again" pile or redesigned. Unless it was a unanimous vote that the meal was awesome, we always asked the question, "What would make this better?" When a meal rated nine or better among all of us, we knew it was a winner!

Another game was to try to guess the ingredients. We still play this game when we go out to a restaurant and like a particular dish. We will then try to reproduce the same taste in our kitchen. If we bring home leftovers, we will compare it with the dish we've created, just to see what we need to tweak in our recipe. My mother and I will brainstorm possible ingredients we can use as substitutes, do some research on that ingredient, and then try to incorporate it into a recipe to see how it responds in the cooking process. If we find something that works, we create variations that are different enough to tantalize the taste buds but not cause us to reinvent the recipe. Each of us, including my son, provide feedback and suggestions based on our own individual preferences.

Accept who you are! You are wonderfully unique, even if you have siblings who were born on the same day as you. There has never been another person exactly like you nor will there ever be! Find ways to love who you have become and who you will be, even with all of your imperfections. Sometimes it's the imperfections that make us beautiful! This includes loving yourself, even in the midst of your struggles. Food restrictions are not the sum of who you are.

Think about how healthy (or unhealthy) you feel at this very moment. You are beginning a wonderful journey toward feeling better and helping your body heal. Take a minute to imagine how much stronger and healthier you will be when you've made positive changes in your life. Keep this model in your mind every time you get frustrated or bored with your options. You are exceptional and you will overcome!

Get back to basics. What is it that you love to do? What motivates and energizes you? If you don't know, figure out what you absolutely dislike and what drains your energy. Once you've identified those things, look to the opposite to see if that's where your passions are hiding. Find time to do those things you love.

Stay positive! Always try to find the positive side of everything. Dare to see things in a new light. Okay, so you can't eat some of your favorite foods. Give yourself a little time to mourn the loss, but then look at the positive side of the issue and find a way to celebrate the new you. What are the other wonderful options available to you? How good will you feel after staying away from foods that make you sick? Who ever knew that food could taste so good? Is this a good excuse to get one of those kitchen gadgets you've been thinking about buying for the last six months? What will you reward yourself with when you meet your goal?

No matter what is going on inside you or around you, practice the art of positive thinking and watch how your health will improve (And so will your cooking!). Situations that once seemed hopeless will become opportunities for success. Don't fret if you try something new and it turns out to be a "failure." Some of our best recipes were "failures" intended to be something else! Besides, you may be just one step away from success. There were some dishes we threw away several times because they were absolutely horrible. In fact, I wouldn't have fed it to the dog, if we had one, but through persistence and the process of elimination, we finally got it right!

Seek out support! Eating differently is a lifestyle change. You are not alone in this effort—many people have had to make this change, just like you. Look at your immediate family and the style in which your family deals with problems. Is your family unit like the Three Musketeers: one for all and all for one? Or is your family more like independent superheroes: every man for himself? Adapt and adjust to find the support you need.

Do any of your friends or co-workers struggle with the same issues? Food is a wonderful way to connect with others. Bring in your favorite healthy recipe to that potluck lunch or going away party and see what happens. I once brought in the granola from this cookbook to a going away party at work. Several months later, people were still talking about how good it was and a couple of people even asked for the recipe! I've used my multiple food allergies as an icebreaker in a conversation with people I've just met. Doors of support and encouragement open up when two people share a hardship.

Look for formal or informal support groups. These can be found in local papers or newsletters, clinics or even on-line. If you can't find one in your area, start one!

Give back to the community and encourage others! Research your illness or allergy and learn as much as you can about it. Share what you've learned. It's empowering! When you talk and share with others, listen to what they are saying and encourage them to share what they know. Everyone has something to contribute. Even those people who are great in their fields of expertise have stood on the shoulders of those who came before them. Build each other up so that you are stronger together.

And this is just the beginning!

Perseverance through hardship builds character and so does the joy and celebration of a new life! There is more awareness now about food sensitivities and intolerances than there were ten years ago—even five. Because of this, more alternative foods are available each year. Take advantage of all your resources and go for it! You have nothing to lose and everything to gain! We are right beside you, cheering you every step of the way!

Kris

The Beginning of June's Journey

I am constantly amazed that a single event in my life can turn my world upside down. By choice, I was a vegetarian, happily living alone in Massachusetts with my two cats in a beautiful apartment. I had an excellent job, a modest 401k, friends, a life routine I loved and traveled whenever I could. Although I didn't know it at the time, this gluten-free journey for me began with a desperate phone call from Kris asking me to move in with her, her new husband, Bob, and my six-year-old grandson, Jonathan.

Bob was ill with a number of disorders, most of which went officially undiagnosed, and, within months of the onset, the combination of illnesses proved to be debilitating. Kris dearly needed another pair of hands with a driver's license. She struggled to simply work a 40-hour week to maintain her job and pay the bills, and I am still amazed she survived on four to five hours of sleep per night.

It took a few months for obligations and employment to fall into place to allow me to move, but as always happens when it's God's idea, events converge in perfect timing. My job ended suddenly when my boss moved his small office into his home, and the race was on to dispose of most of my possessions and pack the rest for moving in two month's time. I was eager to begin my new life, but little did I know the exciting direction it would take me.

I had never lived with a disabled person, and had no idea that by necessity, the entire household must revolve around the needs of that person. We established early on that any changes we made in diet would be for all of us. As a family, we all needed to be supportive of each other and primarily Bob.

In the first month living with Bob, Kris, and Jonathan, I realized being the only vegetarian in the family simply wasn't going to work. I was exhausted after one week of making two meals for every meal and quickly relearned the joys of eating meat and fish. That opened up a whole new culinary world to me and I embraced the changes with joy. I became the head chef in the house to allow Kris more time to care for Bob, which demanded increasing blocks of her time. It also freed her up to research his symptoms and eventually diagnose what doctors were unwilling or unable to do.

It has been my experience that physicians are educated to treat one ailment at a time and tend to ignore what they don't understand, rarely treating the whole body as the interactive miraculous unit it is. As Bob struggled with disabling pain and movement, Kris took on the task of sorting through the tremendous amounts of information in books and the internet for the changes we could make that would give Bob better quality of life. It was a gradual process of elimination as we discovered his many allergies, but with each new change that made a difference for him, we were encouraged. Elimination of artificial sweeteners, certain vegetables, chemical ingredients and eventually gluten brought a measure of relief to some symptoms, but any improvement truly seemed like a drop in the bucket.

By the time we determined Bob was Celiac, Kris noted the correlation to her own body and discovered she too was Celiac. At this point, we had eliminated gluten in all forms, artificial sugars, ginger, peanuts, and tree nuts. As we tried to deal with these new restrictions, Bob's diseases accelerated and, after two weeks in intensive care, he died.

What began as a journey to benefit Bob, became a life-saving way of life for Kris. She carefully monitored her ever-changing body symptoms and continued to try to make sense of the puzzle pieces it presented. We systematically re-engineered our favorite recipes, discovered new ones that delighted our palates, and, just when we thought we had things figured out, Kris began a gradual decline in her overall health due to an elevation of digestive problems. More research revealed she also suffered from Candida, a yeast imbalance, and we were faced with an additional new list of dietary restrictions, which included elimination of tomatoes, anything fermented, soy, fruit, condiments, dairy, natural sugars and yeast. Kris began tracking what she ate and her body's reactions, which revealed further allergies of sorghum, corn in its whole state, and chia seeds.

The impact on Kris was heavy and my heart ached for her. She not only felt physically ill and perpetually exhausted during a time of grieving for the love of her life, but was also faced with a discouragingly limited list of foods she could eat. There were no packaged foods we could fix so we made everything from scratch, which consumed more time than we had. The conversion of recipes and experimentation with combinations of sweeteners like vegetable glycerine and liquid stevia was not only exciting but time consuming. We now had to plan our lives around food preparation and eating.

It was at this time, we realized Jonathan, my grandson, was experiencing many of the same symptoms Kris had, and we determined he was either gluten intolerant or also Celiac. Further analysis and trial and error revealed he had Candida and an allergy to soy. There were more than a few tears from both Kris and Jonathan with the discouragement they both felt. While I didn't experience any of their symptoms, I knew it would take all three of us working together to get both Jon and Kris back to good health.

We proceeded in a logical manner by taking so many fieldtrips to the bookstore that they addressed us by name. We found an endless supply of gluten-free cookbooks and some that even covered a few more of our allergies. We found some books that offered sugar-free recipes, but none that used sweeteners we could tolerate. We were all on our own here, as there were no cookbooks that covered all our allergies and food restrictions.

The next step was to make a list of the foods we could have, and once again we re-engineered our already heavily altered recipes. By now, none of our recipes held much resemblance to the original. We tried foods new to us and new foods on the market. Creativity kicked into high gear. We made adjustments to ingredients and processes, recorded what worked, and what fed the garbage disposal. We needed as much variety in our diet as we could get, and designing and compiling our recipes was the best way to accomplish that.

Our most difficult challenge was to convert muffins, cakes, and desserts to satisfying gluten free, sugar-free treats. After experimenting with all sweeteners available, we settled on a combination of vegetable glycerine and liquid stevia. Combined in the right proportions, it offers a satisfying level of sweetness with a zero glycemic level. Unfortunately, real sugar has a particular volume and texture we always took for granted in our baked goods for which we now had to compensate. Many times, the flavor and sweetness would be right, but the texture was dry—like a rock—or too moist. Other times, the texture was perfect but the proportion of sweeteners left an unpleasant taste. Each recipe became an opportunity to solve an all-new mystery, and, while I prefer British mysteries, the satisfaction I felt when we got it right was wonderful.

At some point, we realized there had to be many other people facing the trauma of multiple allergies and the daunting task of feeding themselves. Because we believe the wheel should not have to be reinvented, and we didn't want anyone else to needlessly go through the discouragement of charting this new world of food restrictions alone, we're offering delicious, tested recipes within the confines of common food allergies. We think you're going to find great eating within the pages of this book and fresh encouragement as you embrace a new way of living.

June

About Candida

In the battle of Celiac Disease and dealing with its complications and contributing factors, the element of Candida keeps surfacing in research connected to Celiac. In fact, Candida and the damage it does to the body can be an underlying factor in more illnesses than it gets credit for. There's a very good chance you are suffering from Candida, as it goes hand in hand with Celiac Disease and many other conditions.

Donald P. Ellsworth, M.D. is a medical doctor with personal experience with Candida. He witnessed the progressive Candida symptoms in his own body but had no base of knowledge about yeast overgrowth until one of his patients educated him. That started him on a journey not only to better health for himself, but on a mission to educate. He saw that Celiac-related problems are much more common than ever before and concluded from his research that it was due to the overgrowth of Candida in the gastrointestinal tract. The body reacts to both gluten and Candida in the same way by producing antibodies that attack both Candida and gluten. As Dr. Ellsworth says, Candida contains amino acid sequences that are identical or very similar to those found in the Celiac induced immune response. That's why our recipes are designed to avoid the foods that feed Candida.

There's a great deal of information available about Candida albicans stemming from personal experience, and it would be well for you to do your own research to better enable you to seek out treatments that are right for you. Here is some basic information to point you in the right direction.

Candida is otherwise known as Candidiasis. The Centers for Disease Control and Prevention describe it this way: "Candidiasis is a fungal infection caused by yeasts that belong to the genus *Candida*. There are over 20 species of *Candida* yeasts that can cause infection in humans, the most common of which is *Candida albicans*. *Candida* yeasts normally live on the skin and mucous membranes without causing infection; however, overgrowth of these organisms can cause symptoms to develop."

Candida albicans infection can be described as superficial, irregular white patches with a red base (Libonati). This overgrowth of yeast creates such an incredibly wide range of symptoms that the medical community has been slow to recognize its existence and danger. Coupled with the fact that Candida cannot be treated with traditional drugs, it is often overlooked by physicians. Many people have found it necessary to do their own diagnosing and then search out treatments. While we're not qualified to discuss or recommend treatments, we can tell you what Candida feels like in the body and the problems it causes.

Candida is found in everyone's body to some extent, and, for many people, the body's own defenses keep it in check through the good bacteria in the intestinal tract. However, Candida can thrive and invade the body if conditions are right for it to multiply. Those conditions can include damaged or inflamed intestinal lining, lack of good bacteria in the intestinal tract, malnutrition, and a compromised immune system. (Libonati)

The Causes of Candida

There are multiple exposures that can be easily identified and can make conditions right for Candida to grow in our bodies. John E. Humiston, M.D. has written about Candida in terms that are easy for the layperson to understand.

From his clinical experience and research, he describes the exposures that most often cause Candida, listed from most common or frequent to least. "The earlier in life one is exposed, the more frequent the exposure, and the more types of exposure one can identify, the worse the Candida infection will likely be." As an example, a child who had frequent ear infections, received repeated antibiotics, and swam regularly in a chlorinated pool in the backyard growing up, would almost definitely have more Candida symptoms as an adult, rather than a person who seldom received antibiotics during childhood, and swam in fresh water or the ocean.

Antibiotics are at the top of the list. While they kill disease-causing bacteria, antibiotics also kill off the normal, protective bacterial flora throughout the body. Most antibiotics are derived from the chemicals fungi make to protect themselves from bacteria, which is why antibiotics are so effective against bacteria. When all bacteria are destroyed, the fungi is then allowed to proliferate, and there's no way to avoid this outcome.

Repeated exposure to swimming in chlorinated pools. Chlorine is a readily available chemical found in swimming pools and Jacuzzis and is used to kill bacteria and algae. Unfortunately, chlorine also kills the body's normal bacterial flora but does not kill the yeast. The result is yeast growth in and on the body when the competing bacteria are eliminated.

Alcohol beverages. Because alcohol is a fermented product it promotes the growth of yeast in the body, particularly affecting the liver. The liver's function is to filter bacteria, viruses, and toxins out of the blood at the rate of 1.5 liters a minute. Its duty also includes breaking down alcohol so it can be removed from the body, but this magnificent organ is also susceptible to infections and problems from accumulated waste, or if the person ingests more alcohol than the body can process. Regular usage of alcohol encourages a fungal infection of the liver, which interferes with the liver's ability to process what is eaten and drunk, slowing the activity of turning what is consumed into nutrients and energy. In addition to the increased imbalance of yeast in the liver, alcohol has been shown to affect the brain through altering neurotransmitters. The brain then desires more alcohol to rebalance these neurotransmitters, which perpetuates the cycle of damage to the liver.

Regular consumption of Candida-promoting foods. Just as alcohol invites Candida growth, foods that feed Candida can initially be craved, becoming the regular food source for a growing and deepening Candida infection. Foods most often craved are coffee, sugar, chocolate, bread, dairy products, vinegar, pickles, tree nuts, peanuts, and sweet fruits such as apples, grapes and bananas. Hormones and antibiotics introduced into our meats and dairy also contribute to Candida overgrowth.

Alcoholism in either parent ups the ante. Alcoholic parents of young children will unknowingly share fungal flora through normal contact with their children. Because they themselves crave Candida-promoting foods, their children's diets will likely contain more of those foods. To a greater extent, Candida problems are observed more often in children of alcoholic parents than non-alcoholic parents.

Birth control hormones. During childbearing years, a woman's body produces a carefully orchestrated pattern of estrogen and progesterone, hormones that produce fertility and menstruation. When birth control hormones are introduced in any form, the secretion pattern is completely altered through providing a steady level of hormone, which prevents eggs from being released by the ovaries. This unnaturally even level of hormone promotes fungal growth.

Mother was always ill. A mother has intimate contact with her child from birth through early childhood. When that mother's immune system is compromised, as evidenced by numerous illnesses, her health has likely been affected by Candida overgrowth, either as a cause or consequence of the illnesses. It would be natural for the mother to unintentionally share this excess fungus with her child. But you cannot blame your mother! The true issue is a lack of understanding of this invasive problem and the chemicals and substances that cause it in our everyday world.

Consistent exposure to mold. Regular exposure to mold on a long-term basis suppresses the immune system and gradually, but surely, establishes a fungal overgrowth in the body. Inhaling mold spores for several hours on a regular basis, such as sleeping in a room with a mold problem, is especially dangerous, made more so by previous exposures such as antibiotics or chlorine. Mold in a home is most often caused by a constant leak in plumbing or a one-time flood experience that was not properly handled. Within a couple of days, mold establishes and grows in carpets, floors and walls, constantly sending spores into the air. If a moldy smell is detected or black mold is visible, you can be sure there is a significant mold problem, but mold may not be that obvious. If you live in an ocean beach community or a coastal area that is frequently overcast, the effects of a constantly wet environment should be considered.

Mercury and mercury fillings also known as silver amalgam fillings. Amalgam was first introduced in the United States in 1830, but was rejected by organized dentistry because of concerns about mercury poisoning. In 1859 the American Dental Association was formed and approved the use of amalgam fillings. The ADA and the Federal Drug Administration still approve its use despite the research and the fact that Norway, Sweden, and Denmark have banned the substance. Dental silver fillings are about 50% mercury by weight and research has proved that mercury vapors are released into the body from chewing action. As a result, mercury enters the digestive system and other body tissues. Mercury has antibacterial, fungal-friendly effects and promotes the growth of yeast wherever it resides in the body. Up until 1999, mercury was used as an antibacterial preservative in vaccines, which appears to also contribute to yeast overgrowth.

Common use of corticosteroids. Corticosteroids are man-made drugs that closely resemble cortisol, a natural hormone secreted by the adrenal glands. Names for this category of drugs are prednisone, hydrocortisone, dexamethasone, and fluticasone along with pretty much any name ending in -lone, -sone, -cort or -ase. You will find them in the forms of inhalers, pills, injections, or creams and primarily used to curb inflammation of allergies, skin rashes, asthma, joint pain, psoriasis, poison ivy and oak, autoimmune diseases as well as many other conditions. Unfortunately, they switch off the body's normal immune reactions, leaving the person vulnerable to the growth of fungi and other microbes. If you read the side effects of the drugs, you will see fungal infections listed.

Exposure to pesticides. Pesticides came into common use in agriculture and even homes after World War II, with DDT being the most popular because of its low cost and effectiveness. Much research has been done on pesticides and their effect on the environment, especially when they enter the water supply. Since the primary purpose of pesticides is to inhibit growth of specific organisms, it appears when they enter the body, they continue on their mission of inhibiting normal flora. Individuals, who had significant exposure, especially as children whether living on former farmland or being directly exposed, can trace Candida symptoms directly to this exposure (Humiston. Candida risk factors).

The Body's Natural Protection

Dr. Humiston goes on to explain that when our bodies are in a healthy state, they have natural protection against Candida in the form of *bacterial flora* and a type of white blood cells called *neutrophils.*

Bacterial flora are microorganisms that live in any area of your body that is not sterile, such as the skin, genital areas, ears, nose, mouth, throat, esophagus, and most of the intestines. In a healthy body, specific bacterial types will populate parts of the body in harmonious existence. Without bacterial flora, undesirable microbes can invade and grow creating a yeast overgrowth, viruses or more serious diseases.

About.com defines neutrophils as a type of white blood cell, produced in the bone marrow and circulated in the blood. Neutrophils are prolific and make up about 50% to 75% of the white blood cells. They respond to infection and attack bacteria and other foreign invaders in a direct way. They are, in fact, the first type of immune cell to arrive at the site of infection, often within an hour. Neutrophils are not limited to working inside the body but will work on the skin surface also. Pus, which is one visible sign of skin infection, contains mainly dead neutrophils, bacteria and cells.

Candida overgrowth occurs when the immune system is suppressed, bacterial flora are killed, and neutrophils are reduced or sluggish. When conditions are right for Candida to grow and the body consumes food such as fermented products, sugars, and anything with "malt" in its name, the expansion of Candida can be significant. It has been estimated that the majority of the population in the industrialized world has yeast overgrowth.

What Happens in the Body

Dr. Humiston explains the progression of Candida overgrowth and how it affects the body:

Candida overgrowth begins in the body due to contact with harmful chemicals, antibiotics, and other substances that suppress the natural immunity or provide food for fungi.

Candida invasion of organs begins affecting the liver to a large extent. Candida usually begins in the intestines. It should be noted that the liver directly receives a large blood supply directly from the intestines, moving Candida throughout the system.

Changes in the liver affect appetite. While it appears there has been no definitive and exhaustive scientific research done specifically to prove that the liver can determine what foods and substances the body desires, Dr. Humiston and others have drawn that conclusion from personal experience and clinical observations. He believes that when Candida takes up residence in the liver and grows, it chemically influences the appetite. The result is that a person will crave the foods that feed Candida—exactly the foods that should be avoided. Those foods include fermented products (including alcohol in all forms), aged cheeses, chocolate, bread, milk, tree nuts and peanuts, and sweet fruits like grapes, bananas and apples. If a person is seriously affected by Candida, there will be craving for vinegar, salad dressings, ketchup and pickles. Young children under eight years of age will typically crave peanut butter, milk, cheese, yogurt, and macaroni and cheese.

Diet causes Candida to become more deeply entrenched. The body will naturally crave more of the foods that feed Candida, causing further yeast overgrowth, often in an accelerated manner at this point. Candida invades the tissues of the body and even if the diet is altered, Candida will persist unless an effective treatment is undertaken.

Candida symptoms appear. Candida affects primarily the digestive, nervous, and immune systems manifesting numerous symptoms, which can range from annoying to serious. At this point, Candida has probably been developing for ten to thirty years after the initial yeast-promoting exposures, continuing to be fed through diet, medications and environment. Because a bewildering array of symptoms develop gradually, many doctors and patients do not recognize Candida as a real cause of disease.

In Dr. Humiston's clinical experience, a typical patient might develop depression, frequent headaches, sleep problems, fatigue, and/or poor memory around age 35, when the actual cause can be traced back to antibiotics received for ear infections as a young child, chlorine exposure from swimming as an older child, and later being on the high school swim team. (Humiston. Candida infection)

Symptoms of Candida

All sources agree that the symptoms of Candida overgrowth can be extensive and, because they are so commonplace in our society, you may think it's simply normal for everyone to have at least some of the symptoms. Dr. Humiston makes it clear that none of these symptoms are part of normal health. We can become desensitized to the symptoms if many people around us are ill. Multiple symptoms may become *common,* but that doesn't make them *normal.* Many of our everyday illnesses, such as asthma, diabetes, epidemic obesity, chronic fatigue, fibromyalgia, ADD/ADHD, autism, and panic attacks were virtually unheard of before the 1970s. In the 1950s, antibiotics were given out freely. From 1945 on, pesticides have been used on the crops and foods we eat. Chlorinated swimming pools, hormones, and antibiotics given to commercial animals we eat, along with the proliferation of birth control pills, have made conditions favorable for Candida to grow. In the 1990s, barley malt was introduced into nearly every baked food along with high-fructose corn syrup as a sweetener. Both foods feed Candida. (Humiston. Candida symptoms)

Following is a list of symptoms associated with Candida overgrowth, compiled from various sources and personal experience. While you may experience only a few of these symptoms, more than likely you will identify with many. Please see the end of this chapter for the sources and resources.

Mental/Emotional/Nervous System:

- Headaches and migraine headaches
- Depression
- Sleep problems: difficulty falling asleep, or waking up in the middle of the night with a mind that won't calm down (typically between 1 and 3 a.m.)
- Irritability
- Confusion
- Brain fog
- Crying spells
- Poor memory
- Anxiety attacks, panic attacks
- Obsessive-compulsive disorder (OCD)
- Sexual problems: impotence or lack of desire, or excessive sexuality
- Attention deficit, hyperactivity (ADD/ADHD)
- Dizziness
- Numbness
- Feeling of floating or not quite being in your body
- Indecisiveness, difficulty organizing and cleaning messy areas
- Apathy
- Fainting
- Persistent extreme fatigue
- Feelings of rage
- Hallucinations
- Nightmares
- Learning disorders
- Mood swings
- Tingling
- Seizures
- Sleepiness
- Poor coordination

Skin and Hair:

- Skin and nail fungal infections (current or past), including athlete's foot, fungal toenails, ringworm, jock itch
- Skin problems like eczema, rashes, psoriasis, hives, dermatitis
- Body odor
- Prematurely graying hair
- Acne
- Cysts
- Dandruff
- Dryness/oiliness
- Flushing
- Pallor
- Sores/infections

Digestive System:

- Cravings for sugar, chocolate, milk, cheese, vinegar, pickles, alcohol, bread, nuts or fruit
- "Metabolic syndrome" which includes adult-onset diabetes, high cholesterol, or triglycerides, high blood pressure
- "Beer belly," also called truncal obesity: excess weight centered around the abdomen
- Acid reflux/GERD (heartburn)
- Hypoglycemia (low blood sugar)
- Bloating
- Stomach cramps
- Rectal itching
- Constipation and/or diarrhea
- Excessively thin or anorexic/bulimic
- Belching
- Burning sensation
- Gas
- Hunger/thirst
- Nausea
- Indigestion
- Pain
- Rumbling
- Stomach ache
- Soiling
- Vomiting
- Mucus in stool
- Hemorrhoids

Eyes:

- Tinea versicolor or itchy eyelids
- Blurred vision
- Pupils always dilated
- Unusually green eyes, or eye color has turned greenish
- Circles under eyes
- Puffy eyes
- Eye pain
- Red eyes
- Sensitive to light
- Spots/floaters
- Tearing

Ears:

- Earache
- Ear infections
- Extreme sensitivity to sound
- Full/blocked/pressure
- Itching
- Ringing in ears

Nasal:

- Itchy nose
- Nosebleeds
- Chronic post-nasal drip
- Runny nose
- Sinus discomfort/face pain
- Sinusitis
- Sneezing fits
- Stuffy nose/sinus congestion

Throat, Mouth, and Gums:

- Bad metallic taste
- Bad breath
- Canker sores
- Choking
- Sore throat
- Thrush (white coating on tongue)
- Dry lips
- Swollen lower lip
- Cracked tongue
- Hoarse voice
- Increased salivation
- Itching
- Mucus
- Sensitive teeth
- Bleeding gums
- Soreness
- Swelling
- Puffy face
- Tightness in throat/difficulty swallowing pills or food

Respiratory System:

- Chest pain
- Persistent cough
- Mucus in throat
- Hay fever symptoms
- Difficulty in breathing
- Pounding pulse
- Rapid breathing
- Rapid or irregular pulse (heart palpitations)
- Shortness of breath
- Tightness in chest
- Wheezing

Lymph System:

- Swollen, tender glands

Genito/Urinary:

- Bed wetting
- Breast swelling
- Frequent urination
- Impotence
- Loss of libido
- Painful urination
- Urgency to urinate
- Recurring yeast infections
- Recurring UTIs (urinary tract infections)
- Cystitis (inflammation of the bladder)

Immune Disorders:

- Asthma
- Allergies
- Recurring infections--colds, ears, bladder, sinus
- Autoimmune disease (lupus, hypothyroidism, arthritis, others)
- Penicillin allergy
- Sensitivities to food, fragrance and chemicals

Weight Problems:

- Easy gain
- Easy loss
- Fluid retention
- Food aversions
- Food cravings
- Night eating
- Need to gain
- Need to lose

Joints:

- Chronic body pain and/or joint pain
- Red/warm
- Swelling
- Muscle aches and stiffness

Whole Body:

- Fatigue
- Muscle or joint pain, fibromyalgia
- Cold feet, cold hands, sometimes cold nose
- Sweating, especially at night
- Uncomfortable at any temperature
- Generalized swelling
- Low/high blood pressure
- Low body temperature
- Spontaneous bruising
- Sweating
- Aching/pain: neck, back, legs
- Shakiness: neck, back, legs
- Weakness: neck, back, legs
- Persistent low-grade fever

Women's Health Issues:

- Premenstrual syndrome (PMS)
- Endometriosis (chronic pelvic pain)
- Infertility (female)
- Miscarriages
- Toxemia in pregnancy (preeclampsia)
- Menstrual irregularities
- Vaginal discharge
- Vaginal yeast infections

Symptoms seen particularly in children up to about eight-years-old:

- Early allergy to foods like milk
- Infections as a baby
- Child had or has frequent ear infections, tonsillitis, strep throat, or bladder infections, especially if these infections were treated with antibiotics
- Cravings for milk, cheese, yogurt, macaroni and cheese, or peanut butter
- Asthma
- "Drama king" or "drama queen"—complains quite vocally and often
- Autism
- Poor sleep patterns—difficulty going to sleep, sleeps too lightly or has frequent nightmares, and wakes up too early (or sometimes too late)
- Too thin or overweight
- Attention deficit with or without hyperactivity (ADD/ADHD)
- Aggressive, poor social interactions, can't stop moving, frequent fights/arguments, or frequent crying
- Pale complexion, dark circles under the eyes

Dr. Humiston is careful to point out that while all of the symptoms listed are definitely seen in Candida patients, and there is evidence that Candida causes or strongly contributes to the development of these problems, Candida may not be the only culprit. Metal toxicity (often mercury), consistent excessive electromagnetic field exposure, and underlying viral infections and petrochemical exposure may cause some of the same symptoms. Treatment for Candida alone will usually bring about significant improvement in symptoms, but further treatments may be necessary to restore health. Support aimed at improving liver, adrenal or thyroid function, or correcting immune and allergy problems may be necessary.

Why Doctors Aren't Getting With The Program

With all this evidence of Candida and the long-term damage it can do, you may be wondering why medical doctors are not more knowledgeable about this serious health risk. Dr. Humiston addresses this question from his own personal professional experience. He says, in medical school and family practice, he was taught that Candida could be damaging only in those patients whose immune systems were severely compromised, such as those with terminal cancer or AIDS patients, which is not true.

He goes on to explain the reasons why Candida is not acknowledged by most physicians:

1. **The myriad of Candida symptoms develop over time, often 10 to 30 years.** Most doctors are not trained to look for evidence of Candida, so they miss the big picture. In medicine, doctors tend to look at diseases and symptoms in a singular manner, dealing with one symptom at a time, one disorder at a time, and ignore the interconnectedness of symptoms. This oversimplified approach to disease impedes the physician's understanding of a complex disease such as Candida with its multiple symptoms in various organ systems. Numerous symptoms that progress gradually will appear to be unrelated to a doctor untrained in the complexities of Candida.
2. **Candida is so widespread that your own doctor probably has it and doesn't know.** If your doctor has record of you experiencing similar symptoms but he or she is not familiar with the complexities of Candida, you will not be accurately diagnosed. When so many people have similar symptoms, it's more difficult for doctors to think of those symptoms as abnormal, especially without a single defining identifying symptom.
3. **At present, reliable lab tests to diagnose Candida do not exist.** Candida grows through forming tentacles around cells rather than moving loosely through the blood, so standard or even invasive medical tests cannot accurately report the extent of Candida growth, even though Candida can be seen in biopsies. Clinical diagnosis through assessing the exposures and counting up the symptoms is the only diagnostic tool available. It should be noted that other diseases such as Parkinson's disease, mental illness, and migraine headaches are diagnosed in this same manner.
4. **Eradication of Candida is very difficult, and almost none of the treatments are effective, including prescription drugs and over-the-counter treatments.** The medical community, and even many patients, are resistant to embracing any treatments aside from prescription drugs, and without an effective treatment for Candida, physicians have little interest in educating themselves or patients about this disorder. There are particular medical properties found in nature that cannot be accurately synthesized in a laboratory, which means drug manufacturers are neither interested in the research into this disorder nor the search for effective treatments.

5. **Standard medical diagnostics and treatment is focused on treating the symptoms, not correction of the underlying cause.** Unfortunately, simply treating the symptoms of Candida will bring temporary improvement, but lasting effects will not be achieved until the fungus is killed.
6. **Doctors are afraid to do what other doctors are not doing.** Recognizing and treating Candida falls outside the comfort zone of the medical community and requires courage and innovative thinking. Most physicians are not willing to open themselves to criticism even if current methods of treatment are ineffective.
7. **Candida is not a high-profile disorder so finding relevant information for doctors is difficult.** Many doctors rely on medical journals as their main or even sole source of keeping abreast of medical advancements. It is unfortunate that the large volume of published studies appearing regularly in medical journals are statistical comparisons of patented drugs, sponsored by drug manufacturers, and almost nothing of new, innovative ways to treat disease is being published, especially if it has to do with natural substances. Medical journals cannot afford to lose the advertising revenues from drug manufacturers, which greatly limit their ability to provide any new information of substance. For the same reasons, significant funds are not being set aside for research on Candida. Much of the information available has come from individuals and professionals with personal experience with Candida. (Humiston. Candida and the medical profession)

Treatment of Candida requires diet changes, and many people feel it would be too painful to give up certain foods. This fear is expressed by people who have tried an ineffective program or who are thinking about attempting treatment. In reality, any emotional discomfort or physical craving that is experienced from the elimination of certain Candida-promoting foods is greatly offset by the reduction of symptoms.

The severity of Candida symptoms will vary with each person and the level of infection. For me (June), at the height of my Candida overgrowth, I had an unexplained and persistent low-grade fever that went on for weeks. My body reacted within minutes to anything fermented—especially vinegar, and I could count on immediate gas, bloating, a vaginal itch, and fever.

Another contributing factor to be considered is whether your sexual partner shows any signs of Candida. It is possible to pass Candida back and forth. As a rule, if one of you needs treatment, you both do.

Our goal is not to promote a specific treatment but to simply make you aware of Candida and how it may be affecting your health. At the very least, you can avoid the foods that feed it, and that's why you won't find any dairy products, sugar, artificial sweeteners, sweeteners with a high glycemic value, sugary fruits, tomatoes, yeast, or fermented products in our recipes. The only exceptions are two bread recipes clearly labeled with small amounts of vinegar and yeast.

In this book, we present gluten-free recipes that are satisfying, exciting to your palate, and do not feed Candida. Our recipes are not meant to be a treatment for eradicating Candida but are, instead, simply aimed at diminishing the exposure to foods that feed the fungi. If our recipes spark creativity in you to design your own dishes, then our goals have been doubly met.

Works Cited

About.com. Neutrophils - What are Neutrophils. About.com Colon Cancer. Retrieved February 12, 2013 from http://coloncancer.about.com/od/glossary/g/neutrophils.htm.

Centers for Disease Control and Prevention. (2012). Candidiasis. Retrieved January 13, 2013, from http://www.cdc.gov/fungal/candidiasis/.

Ellsworth, Donald P., M.D. Natural Wellness Choices - The Candida, Celiac, Thyroid Connection. Posted Saturday, December 6, 2008. Retrieved January 26, 2013, from http://naturalwellnesschoices.blogspot.com/2008/12/Candida-celiac-thyroid-connection.html

Gustafson, Helen & O'Shea, Maureen. The Candida Directory & Cookbook. Published by Celestial Arts, 1994. ISBN 978-0-89087-714-2.

Humiston, John E., M.D. Updated: May 11, 2010. CandidaMD, Candida and the medical profession. Retrieved January 10, 2013, from http://www.Candidamd.com/Candida/doctors.html

Humiston, John E., M.D. Updated: May 11, 2010. CandidaMD, Candida infection. Retrieved January 10, 2013, from http://www.Candidamd.com/Candida/getCandida.html

Humiston, John E., M.D. Updated: January 12, 2011. CandidaMD, Candida risk factors. Retrieved January 3, 2013, from http://www.Candidamd.com/Candida/exposures.html

Humiston, John E., M.D. Updated: January 12, 2011. CandidaMD, Candida symptoms. Retrieved January 10, 2013, from http://www.Candidamd.com/Candida/symptoms.html

Libonati, Cleo, RN, BSN on September 10th, 2009. Treating Candida Albicans Intestinal Yeast Overgrowth in Celiac Disease. Retrieved January 11, 2013 from http://glutenfreeworks.com/blog/2009/09/10/treating-Candida-albicans-intestinal-yeast-oevergrowth-in-celiac-disease/#.UPMpDegcSN8

Richards, Lisa. The Candida Diet: Candida Symptoms. Retrieved February 9, 2013 from http://www.theCandidadiet.com/Candidasymptoms.htm pages 3-4.

Subtle Places For Allergens To Hide

As you may have discovered, allergens can hide in the most unlikely places, and even products that have been safe before can have changes in formula. Products often have fillers that are common allergens, such as soy. I admit that there are times when I feel bewildered by ingredient lists. I mean, why is a chemical sweetener (sorbitol) a necessary ingredient in shaving cream?

If your allergies are not severe, you may think a little bit won't hurt you, or if you don't break out in a rash, there's no problem. But the truth is, you may not know what it's doing to your body. Many of the effects of allergens can be subtle but reactions may intensify with multiple symptoms that may leave you back at square one. It's best to be safe and read all labels.

Be especially cognizant of anything that can be absorbed sublingually. When a substance is placed under your tongue, it diffuses through mucous membranes and absorbs into the vast capillary system. As a result, the substance has a fairly direct route into your bloodstream. (Connelly. Why We Take Medicines Under Our Tongue)

This is not an inclusive list by any means, but only meant to jog your brain to think in terms of your own lifestyle and places you might not have thought to look for allergens.

- Suntan lotion
- Shaving cream
- Shampoo
- Hair conditioner
- Hair coloring
- Perm solutions
- Facial cleansers
- Moisturizing lotions
- Foundational makeup
- Eye shadows
- Mascara
- Lash conditioners/thickeners
- Toothpaste
- Mouthwash
- Hair spray
- Household detergents including dish soap
- Prescription medications (ask your pharmacist to see the inactive ingredients)
- Generic drugs as opposed to brand name drugs
- The hard coating encasing pills
- Ingredients used to make gel caps for capsules
- Lotion used in ultrasound (ask in advance and insist on knowing)
- Nonstick cooking sprays
- Spices
- Natural flavorings (that obscure listing at the end of ingredients that can be anything)

- Polishing agents dental hygienists use (insist on knowing--most agents have gluten)
- Body wash
- Fabric softener
- Dryer sheets
- Moist flushable wipes
- Products you've always been able to trust before (because formulas change without notice to the public)
- Laundry detergent
- Toilet paper
- Anything that goes on your body, in your body or can be inhaled

Works Cited

Connelly, Thomas P., D.D.S. printed in The Huffington Post February 18, 2011 08:38 AM. Why We Take Medicines Under Our Tongue. Retrieved January 22, 2013, from http://www.huffingtonpost.com/thomas-p-connelly-dds/medicine-in-the-body-_b_823530.html

Equipment In The Well-Stocked Kitchen

What does a well-stocked kitchen look like? There are probably as many answers as the number of people you ask, and, while answers vary greatly, there are some common denominators.

We find that cooking gluten free for multiple allergies means spending more time in the kitchen, more regularly. When you can't open up a packaged meal or put a frozen dinner in the microwave because you'll get incredibly sick, the alternative is using fresh vegetables and made-from-scratch meals. Cooking in this manner takes more effort, so it's important that your kitchen is set up to maximize your space and time.

I have to admit that before I moved in with Kris, my idea of buying kitchen equipment ran more toward being frugal than practical. Much to my amazement and puzzlement, she came home with multiples of everything and, at first, I thought it was a huge waste of money. However, the more I cooked and baked, the more I realized she was onto something.

What follows is a list of kitchen equipment we find indispensable and why or how we use it. That doesn't mean you have to go out and buy everything on our list. If you've been cooking and baking for some time, you may already have everything you need in your kitchen to function at a high level. This list is only a suggestion; therefore, ultimately, you will have to decide what works for you and your lifestyle, but do read through this section. You may find a new use for some items you already have.

A Great Stand Mixer

This is at the top of our list of important items and probably the most expensive piece of equipment we have. After doing a lot of research, we decided on a Bosch Universal Plus Mixer. It has an 800-watt motor, which means it is powerful enough to do just about anything we need it to do. The mixer bowl latches onto the base and remains stationery while the beaters revolve around the bowl, unlike conventional mixers. It comes with two types of beaters—standard and dough hooks. It is ingeniously designed with a cover that completely seals the top of the mixer bowl—a feature I especially like.

We opted to get a food processor attachment to our Bosch that will chop, slice, and shred at the twist of a button. The bowl part of the unit is smaller and also works perfectly for mixing small amounts that could get lost in the larger mixer bowl.

In addition, the food processor attachment to the Bosch is the only unit we found that grinds seeds and nuts for butters. This is an important staple in our diet, as even the best brands of sunbutter contain some form of sugar, which Kris cannot tolerate. We buy seeds and nuts and make our own butters, which taste far better than any we have found in jars.

Handheld Mixer

Small, handheld mixers are a wonderful invention and can be used in a multitude of situations where a large, stand mixer just won't work. There's no need to search out the most expensive model or brand. One from a discount store will probably last you ten years if you treat it right.

Blender

We use our blender often, and, since we have a separate food processor, we feel no need to buy an exotic or expensive blender. Even the best blender has its limitations, so don't try to use it for something it's not designed to do, like grinding seeds. I admit to being a slow learner and have trashed two blenders that way.

There are two styles of blenders: one has a center piece in the cover that can be removed for pouring liquids directly into the center of the blades, and one with an offset cover. Most of the time, the style makes no difference, unless you're making something like mayonnaise, which requires oil to be poured slowly directly into the center.

Mini Food Processor

I was first introduced to mini food processors when my mother gave me one as a Christmas gift. At that time, I wasn't into cooking and didn't know the difference between a blender and a juicer. Over the years, I realized how useful and easy to use this small appliance was, and continued to use my gift over 20 years until it died. We now have a much newer version and use it for chopping vegetables in a fraction of the time it would take to set up a full-sized food processor. We especially appreciate it for tear-free onion chopping.

Measuring Spoons

There are numerous types and shapes of measuring spoons on the market and not all of them are created equally. The most common are stainless steel spoons that are broad and flat. Another type is often plastic with round, chunky spoons. These all have their use but don't fit well in spice jars, which I find really annoying. Our favorite set is stainless steel with narrow, elongated rectangular spoons that fit well into spice and herb jars. The beauty of these measuring spoons is that a set contains 1/8, 1/4, 1/2, 3/4, 1 teaspoon and 1 tablespoon. We suggest you buy multiple sets of measuring spoons, as there are times when you need a tablespoon measure for a wet ingredient and a tablespoon measure for a dry ingredient in the same recipe.

Wooden Spoons

We keep wooden spoons handy by storing them upright in a small crock on the countertop. We have varying sizes, from oriental soupspoon size to a large bamboo spoon. Most spoons are raw wood or untreated, and require "seasoning" before using. Please refer to the formula for curing wooden utensils in the "How To" section of this book.

Dry Measure Cups

Like measuring spoons, these come in many shapes and configurations. Multiple sets are the key here—we have four sets and never have to stop and wash a cup. Try to get at least one set that has a configuration of 1/4, 1/3, 1/2, 2/3, 3/4, and 1 cup.

Wet Measure Cups

The most common kind you will see is Pyrex in one cup, two cup, four cup, or larger sizes. We have a glass bowl with a handle and markings on the side that holds nine cups and doubles as a mixer bowl. Choose sizes that work for your cooking style, and keep them together in a convenient place.

Strainers

We have multiple strainers in many shapes and sizes. Each one has its usefulness and best purpose, depending on the strainer size and the hole sizes in the strainer. You can find strainers in department stores, high end cooking stores, grocery stores, and even dollar stores, and this is an investment that won't break the bank. Find a variety that suit your needs, and keep them in a handy location in your kitchen.

Splatter Screen

This is a large, flat-screened disk with a handle. The mesh is a tight weave and especially useful for straining washed grains and rices. Quinoa is a tiny grain that slips right through strainers, except for the splatter screen. For this purpose alone, it's worth the small investment. However, since it's made of stainless steel, it's best not to run it through your dishwasher as, in a short time, it may rust.

Rubber Scrapers aka Rubber Spatulas

Of all the things in our kitchen, we use rubber spatulas more than anything else. They come in all sizes and shapes, rigid, soft, short, long, large, small, flat, and contoured. Our mixer bowl came with a rigid spatula specifically designed to fit the bowl's curvature, but, for most purposes, we use small spatulas that are about 3" long on a long handle. Because I generally have my hands full when I realize I need a spatula, we have them conveniently placed on the two counters where we do our mixing. Spatulas are inexpensive items that can be found in a variety of stores, including dollar stores, so stock up with a minimum of 6 to 12.

Rubber spatulas can be run through your dishwasher, and, if the plastic head can be easily removed from the handle, be sure to remove the head before washing. Bacteria and mold can find ways into that area and get pretty ugly.

Garlic Press

This little gadget is an essential item in our kitchen. You'll find several designs in various brands, but they all work about the same way. We have two presses that both hold a large garlic clove and one that will hold several cloves. If you have pain in your hands, go for the smaller size, as the larger press requires a lot of pressing power.

If you are new to cooking with fresh garlic, don't be intimidated. Fresh garlic is so much better than dried or even jarred garlic and is incredibly easy to use with outstanding results. Fresh garlic also stores well at room temperature for several weeks.

Cutting Boards

The number and type of cutting boards you choose depends on your personal preference for cutting surfaces, availability of storage space, whether it fits into your dishwasher, counter space, and probably a few other factors I haven't mentioned. We have various sizes of wooden boards, hard plastic boards, and, my favorite, a large piece of Corian I bought at a flea market from a vendor who made them out of the cutouts from kitchen counters. My next favorite is a rigid plastic board that has a fairly large surface but still fits in the dishwasher.

You will need a minimum of two boards. When making a meal that has meat, poultry or fish, be sure to use a separate board for cutting vegetables to avoid cross contamination of bacteria.

Wooden boards are generally purchased as raw wood and need to be treated or "seasoned" before use. If you buy the best boards and treat them well, you'll be able to pass them down to your grandchildren.

If you or your spouse are handy in the workshop and plan to make your own cutting boards, choose your wood carefully. Tightly grained hardwoods with small pores such as birch, maple, walnut, beech, mahogany, or cherry are best for reducing scoring of the cutting surface and absorption of liquid and bacteria into the surface. Although oak is a hardwood, it has large pores that retain bacteria, even after washing, making it a poor choice for this purpose. (Baylor) (Allen)

Teak, however, "offers a unique combination of functionality, elegance, and carefree maintenance. Teak wood boasts a naturally high level of oily resins, which gives the hardwood its trademark ability to repel moisture, warping, and other signs of aging." (Proteak)

Although bamboo is technically a grass and "not a tree, it grows at a much quicker rate than any other wood. From start to harvest (60 to 70 feet tall), it can take just four years. Bamboo is naturally anti-microbial, therefore stopping bacteria from growing. It is also one of the strongest yet lightest materials around. Bamboo is 16% stronger than Maple and is 33% lighter in weight than Oak." (Core Bamboo)

Do some research and select wood with care, especially if are using a tropical hardwood, as some species contain toxins or allergens. In any case, refer to the formula for curing wooden utensils in the "How To" section to make wooden items last forever.

Mini Muffin Pans

Mini muffin pans are great for making candies. Thankfully, there are also mini muffin papers to be found in most grocery stores. Invest in a set of nonstick pans and resist the urge to run them through the dishwasher. It degrades the finish and causes rust.

Standard Muffin Pans

Good nonstick muffin pans are a must, and, unless you bake for a troop, two pans that will result in two dozen muffins should work. It pays to invest in good muffin pans and then treat them with respect. Never run muffin pans through the dishwasher, and be careful not to scratch the surface of the pans with metal utensils.

Be sure to read the small print on the packaging on your new muffin pan as well. I ruined a pan by using commercial nonstick spray, not realizing it would remove the finish, which is a good reason to use oil instead. If nonstick spray can mess up my favorite muffin pan, it can't be good for a fragile body.

Muffin Paper Liners

Muffin paper liners are found in grocery stores. Keep a supply on hand, and use them liberally for anything you want to come out of a muffin pan easily. We always grease papers before filling them, but, even so, we have discovered that some breads and cakes will stick to the papers when hot but are completely "peelable" when the baked goods are cooled. These make clean up so much easier and allow baked goods to be easily carried in a lunch box.

Misto® Oil Sprayer

At one point, there was only one store brand of nonstick spray that did not have soy in it. Not too many months later, the manufacturer changed the formula and we could no longer use it without Kris and Jonathan getting sick. A reasonable alternative is a Misto Oil Sprayer. Fill the brushed steel canister with your favorite oil, pump the lid, and spray on pans to prevent sticking. We have one for olive oil and one for canola.

Cutlery Set

A set of good cutlery is essential if you're going to spend quality time in your kitchen, or if you want to spend less time in your kitchen. There are many great brands, and prices range from inexpensive to chef's grade quality that will make a serious dent in your 401k. The key to choosing knives is in how they feel in your hand. Go to a good cooking store and talk with a salesperson that knows about knives. He or she can guide you into the best choice. When you put the knife in your hand, it should feel like an extension of your hand, and not an awkward intruder.

Some knife sets come in a wooden storage block but, if yours doesn't, it's a good investment. Setting the block in a convenient location on your countertop is a great way to store your knives and also helps keep your knives sharp. Turn the cutting block if necessary so knife blades can be inserted horizontally or with the blade up to minimize dulling the knives.

You will need at least one chef's knife: the kind with a curved blade. There's an art to cutting and chopping, and, if you're new to this part of the prep process, watch some real chefs on TV in a good cooking program, or check your local library for a video on using knives. Take note of the ways they use knives and the rocking motion to make accurate cuts. You'll also notice if the knife is being held in the right hand, the left hand holding the food will have fingers curled under and knuckles up. If your fingers are extended flat, you have a greater chance of cutting off a finger or, at the least, wrecking a perfectly good manicured nail.

Rolling Pin

Most rolling pins are wooden, but I have seen beautiful marble rollers. Some are one piece, and others have separate handles that are stationery while the outer part actually does the turning. What you choose will be your own personal preference. Base your choice on how it feels in your hands. Kris prefers a one-piece roller, but I find that type clumsy to use. We use a rolling pin for rolling out pie crusts, an occasional cookie dough, or crushing chips or cookies into crumbs.

Spray Bottle

Any inexpensive type will do, but keep it dedicated for clean kitchen use. We spritz the counter top when we need to put down waxed paper or plastic wrap to make the wrap stay in place.

Storage Containers That Fit Nicely Into Your Cupboards

When we began stocking our kitchen with new flours and ingredients that frequently came in non-resealable plastic bags, we quickly realized we needed containers that would fit into our available space. As we increased our stash of new ingredients, we moved our containers several times until we found cupboards that were convenient and large enough to store like ingredients together. Organization that works for you is the key here. Common physics told us that round containers left too much wasted space, so we chose plastic square or rectangular containers in 8 cup and 9 1/2 cup sizes. The lids seal to keep out moisture, and the containers can be labeled.

It is super important that you label everything, as there are several flours that look alike, and you're not going to remember what you have. Put the labels on the front and/or top of the container and be sure to mark it GF, especially if you have non-GF ingredients in the house. It's impossible to tell the difference from GF and non-GF oatmeal, for example.

Dorm Sized Refrigerator

There are some ingredients that should be refrigerated, so, if you have the room for a dorm-sized fridge, this is a good investment. For those items that need refrigeration to extend shelf life, indicate that refrigeration is needed in some way on the label that makes sense to you. For example, our coconut and potato flours have brightly colored labels so we know at a glance where to return them. This may not seem important, but when you are doing a recipe with 8 different containers that all look alike, you do not want to stop to research the internet to see if the bean flour or the coconut flour was the one that had to be refrigerated.

Labels

We recommend labeling all containers to cut down on search time and errors. You may think this is a waste of time, but you'll be glad you did this the first time you try to figure out whether you have cornstarch, arrowroot starch, potato starch, or tapioca flour in hand. We use blank address labels and blue painter's tape for the containers that labels won't stick to.

Four-Sided Grater

We recommend a four-sided grater, also known as a box grater, because of ease of use and the stability of four points on a surface. There is much less chance of raking your knuckles over the sharp points if your grater is firmly planted. Buy one made of stainless steel for a moderate price.

Parchment Paper

Parchment paper is used to line baking pans for anything you absolutely don't want to stick to the pan. Cream puffs are a good candidate for parchment paper. You can purchase parchment in most grocery stores, and it's a great item to have on hand.

Citrus Juicer

We started out with a small electric citrus juicer, and, when we wore that out, we tossed the base and now use just the top part, which works fine manually. Your great-grandmother didn't have electricity and she was able to make lemonade using a glass citrus juicer. Check out what's available in your area, gauge how much you will use it, calculate your budget, and make your choice as to what works best for you.

Vegetable Peelers

We both love the great variety of vegetable peelers on the market. Some blades are made of stainless steel, some of super sharp porcelain. Some have ergonomic padded handles and others are just functional. One of my favorites is designed for thin peels like carrots but doesn't work well for vegetables with thick peelings, like winter squash. One peeler we have has sharp "teeth" in the blade that only work on thick-skinned vegetables. Buy a variety of peelers and decide which ones work best for you. Eventually they dull and have to be tossed, but, by that time, you'll know which you want to replace and which you are most likely to use only in a pinch.

Stockpot

This is a large, stainless steel pot frequently used in canning. No, we're not suggesting you go back to nature and take up canning, but you can easily make your own beef, vegetable, and chicken broths. We try very hard not to waste anything, and all our vegetable peelings, parsley stems, celery tops, sweet pepper insides, spinach stems, onion, shallot, and garlic skins go into sealable gallon bags in the freezer. We pour off liquids from steamed and boiled vegetables, as well as canned vegetables, and freeze these for broth bases. When we have at least four gallon bags of vegetable peelings, we cook up a batch of broth and store it in labeled, serving sized freezer containers. These keep for months when frozen. You'll see recipes for the various broths we use under the section for "Mixes."

Resealable Plastic Bags

I personally believe resealable plastic bags are the greatest invention since the toaster. We frequently make up multiple batches of mixes, such as the dry ingredients for Burger Buns, or anything we bake often, and store them in plastic bags—labeled of course. Gallon bags get filled with vegetable scraps and peelings and are stored in the freezer for broth to be made at a later time. Snack bags are just the right size for portioning out lunchbox snacks. Sandwich bags will also hold half an onion in the refrigerator for later use. Buy every size you can find from snack bags to gallon size, and use them liberally.

Permanent Marker

Get at least one fine point permanent marker for labeling purposes. We suggest you don't write directly on reusable containers. You can write directly on plastic bags, but for bags that go into the freezer, writing eventually comes off. It's best to put a label on these items.

Funnels

Funnels come in many different sizes and each has its own usefulness. The most economical funnels are made of plastic and can be found in 1/4", 3/8" and, my favorite, 1" size. You can find them in grocery stores, dollar stores, hardware stores, and automotive stores. The 1" size is sold most often in the automotive and parts section and is typically marketed for putting oil into a car. Buy as many sizes as you can find, nest them together, and store them in one place. You'll be surprised how many times you will use funnels, especially if you buy certain products in bulk.

Electric Rice Cooker

One of the neat things about being in the military is that you get to meet so many wonderful people. An Asian wife introduced me to the necessity of a good rice cooker. Choose the best size for how you will use it. If you are going to entertain friends, you will want a larger one than if you're going to serve two. If you get one with a steamer tray on top, you can also use it to steam veggies. Follow manufacturing or food preparation instructions for the food you are cooking.

Food Scale (preferably digital)

We use our scale often in weighing out meat portions, pasta if we're not using the whole box, or to determine how many potatoes in a pound for a recipe. British and Canadian recipes list ingredients by weight, mostly in grams, so it's important to find a scale that shows both ounces and grams. While this is not a must-have, if you have one, you will use it more often than expected.

We tried using a good postage scale and, after an embarrassing encounter with the man in the meat section who had to prove to me the packaged meat weighed out accurately, we realized the postage scale's abilities were limited to envelopes under 16 ounces and Cub Scout Pinewood Derby cars.

Food Scooper Thing

We consider this item essential in our kitchen. It is known by several names, depending on the brand—Bash, Chop and Scoop Cutter (quite descriptive), Food Scoop, Tools Bench Scrape Shovel (sounds like it should be stored in the garage), and Multi-Purpose Pastry Scraper/Chopper or simply Scraper/Chopper. It's usually a 4 1/2" x 6" stainless steel flat utensil that allows you to scoop food up off a cutting board. We have two and use them every day.

Baking Dishes

We prefer ovenproof glass baking dishes in 8" x 8" size and 8" x 11" size. Buy the least expensive ones you can find at discount stores and dollar stores.

There are endless shapes and sizes of baking dishes and casserole dishes. If you're new to cooking and baking, it will become obvious to you quickly which sizes and shapes you will use the most.

Baking Pans

We prefer the nonstick kind and wash them by hand to preserve the finish. Choose sizes that make sense for the way you do things and treat them well. Be sure to read the instructions for your pans to make them last longer, and, if they're nonstick, do not put them in the dishwasher! You won't notice at first, but the dishwasher liquid immediately begins to degrade the finish.

Bread Pans

We have two nonstick finish standard sized bread pans (5" x 9") but rarely use them both at the same time. To make foods come out of them easier, I always line bread pans with aluminum foil, but not everyone will find this necessary.

We also have smaller bread pans, 3 1/2" x 7" and even smaller silicone pans 2 1/2" x 4 1/2". Buy what works for you and the way you bake.

Cookie Sheets

It pays to invest in a good brand of cookie sheets, preferably nonstick. They need to be heavy enough so they don't go "wonky" in a hot oven and keep the finish intact. The kind you see in the grocery store are usable in a pinch but, if you can afford the good stuff, you'll be glad you made the investment.

The large sized cookie sheet measures 11" x 17" and the usual size for the smaller variety is 9" x 16". Lately, I've been covering them with aluminum foil before use to aid in cleanup.

Cooling Racks

Stainless steel wire cooling racks are essential if you make muffins, cookies, crackers, or just need to allow a pan to cool, and we suggest buying three. You can find them at dollar stores and discount stores, but choose racks that have a square weave, as opposed to long wires that allow cookies and crackers to fall through.

I have seen nonstick coating on wire racks and, personally, I think it's just another attractive attempt to separate me from my money. I've never had anything stick to a wire rack that couldn't be easily taken care of in the dishwasher.

Electric Ice Cream Maker

For most people, this is not a must-have item, but for us it is. We love ice cream and always have some we have made in our freezer. The flavor possibilities are countless, and homemade ice cream is much more economical that gluten free, allergy-free brands.

We have two small, electric ice cream makers that produce up to 4 cups of ice cream each, allowing us to have two different flavors going at once. Look for the least expensive brand you can find and you'll be happy with the results.

Works Cited

Allen, Eric. "Build and Keep a Cutting Board, a tutorial from Nils Wessel of Brooklyn Butcher Blocks." Web. http://kaufmann-mercantile.com/how-to-build-and-maintain-a-cutting-board/. Retrieved February 4, 2013.

Baylor, Chris, Woodworking Guide for About.com. "Make a Hardwood Cutting Board." Web. http://woodworking.about.com/od/woodworkingplansdesigns/ss/CuttingBoard.htm. Retrieved February 4, 2013.

Core Bamboo. "Why Bamboo?" Web. http://www.corebamboo.com/whybamboo/. Retrieved February 4, 2013.

Proteak Renewable Forestry. Web. http://www.proteak.com/. Retrieved February 4, 2013.

Food Shopping List To Stock Your Cupboards

If you are new to gluten free, sugar-free cooking for multiple allergies, the whole concept can be overwhelming. Our goal is to break it all down into segments that are easier to deal with, one at a time. One of those segments is about stocking your cupboards with items likely to be used most.

For your convenience, we have made a list of the flours we reach for most often. As you figure out what works for you and what doesn't, you'll also learn how to save money on your purchases. For example, we buy vegetable glycerine by the gallon through the internet, which is more cost effective than buying at our local health food store.

Check your local oriental market for anything on this list that they may carry. You'll find white rice flour there but probably not brown rice flour. Cornstarch and tapioca flour are fairly easy to locate as well, but arrowroot starch will most likely need to be purchased from a local health food store. Take notes on where you find products until shopping in this new way becomes second nature to you.

Be sure to read the section on "Storage Containers That Fit Nicely In Your Cupboard" under "Equipment In The Well Stocked Kitchen" for more helpful information.

Flours We Use Most:

- White Rice Flour
- Tapioca Flour aka Starch
- Bean Flour aka Gram, Garfava, Garbanzo or Chickpea
- Arrowroot Starch aka Flour aka Powder
- Potato Starch (not Potato Flour)
- Brown Rice Flour
- Xanthan Gum
- Cornstarch

Flours That Need To Be Refrigerated:

- Potato Flour (not Potato Starch)
- Coconut Flour
- Corn Flour (not Cornmeal or Masa Harina)

Product Brands

As we sorted through the many products available in stores and online that met our criteria for gluten free and sugar free, we made a list of the products we used. It's important to read the ingredients, and be certain products are not processed on equipment shared with products to which you may be allergic.

Not all products are available in all areas of the country, and you may have access to brands we're not familiar with. This list will give you points of reference, if you need to seek out more choices than available to you locally.

At this printing, these products are safe for us, but do your own research. Products can change without notice.

Product, Brand and Website

Alcohol-Free Extracts/Flavorings - Frontier - www.frontiercoop.com
Apricot Kernel Oil - Spectrum Naturals - www.spectrumorganics.com
Black Cherry Concentrate - Lakewood Organic - www.lakewoodjuices.com
Brown Rice Syrup - Lundberg Family Farms - www.lundberg.com
Browning & Seasoning Sauce - Kitchen Bouquet - www.chloroxprofessionals.com
Buttery Spread - Earth Balance - www.earthbalancenatural.com
Cacao Nibs - Navitas Naturals - www.navitasnaturals.com
Coconut Flakes (unsweetened) - My Spice Sage - www.myspicesage.com
Coconut Flakes (unsweetened) - Let's Do...Organic - www.edwardandsons.com
Coconut Flour - Let's Do...Organic - www.edwardandsons.com
Coconut Flour - Bob's Red Mill - www.bobsredmill.com
Coconut Milk and Cream - Aroy-D - www.thaiagri.com
Coconut Oil - Dr. Bronner's - www.serendipol.com
Cocoa Powder - Hershey's - www.hersheys.com
Coconut Nectar - Coconut Secret - www.coconutsecret.com
Coconut Sugar - Madhava - www.madhavasweeteners.com
Coconut Sugar - Wholesome Sweeteners, Inc. - www.organicsugars.biz

Cranberry Concentrate - Lakewood Organic - www.lakewoodjuices.com

Daiya Vegan Cheese - Daiya - www.daiyafoods.comn

Flaxseed (ground) - Bob's Red Mill - www.bobsredmill.com/gluten-free

Flaxseed (ground) - Spectrum Essentials - www.spectrumorganics.com

Green Olives without vinegar - Mediterranean Organic - www.mediterraneanorganic.com

Hash Browns (Baby Cakes & Smiley Fries) - McCain - www.mccainpotatoes.com

Hemp Hearts - Manitoba Harvest - www.manitobaharvest.com

Liquid Stevia - SweetLeaf - www.SweetLeaf.com

Maca Powder - Navitas Naturals - www.navitasnaturals.com

Mochi - Grainaissance - www.grainaissance.com

No-Salt Seasoning - Kirkland - www.costco.com

Oatmeal Cream - Hill Estates - www.creamhillestates.com

Oatmeal - Bob's Red Mill - www.bobsredmill.com/gluten-free

Pasta - Seitenbacher - www.seitenbacher.com

Perfect Pinch Salt Free - Seasoning McCormick - www.perfectpinch.com

Pesto Paste - Amore - www.amorebrand.com

Pine Nuts - Pinyon Penny's - www.pinenut.com

Pizza Crust Mix - Chebe - www.chebe.com

Quinoa Nature's - Earthly Choice - www.earthlychoice.com

Quinoa - TruRoots - www.truroots.com

Quinoa Pasta - Ancient Harvest - www.quinoa.net

Rice Milk - Kirkland - www.costco.com

Rice Milk - Westsoy - www.westsoy.biz

Shortening - Spectrum - www.spectrumorganics.com

Sunflower Lecithin Liquid - Azure Standard - www.azurestandard.com

Sweet Potato Puree - Farmer's Market - www.farmersmarketfoods.com

Tahini - Joyva - www.joyva.com

Tahini - Once Again - www.onceagainnutbutter.com

Tapioca Syrup - John Mountain - www.sweetharvestfoods.com

Tapioca Syrup - Barry Farm - www.barryfarm.com

Vegetable Glycerine - Now Solutions - www.nowfoods.com

Yacon Powder - Ojio - www.myojio.com

Yacon Powder - Navitas Naturals - www.navitasnaturals.com

Yacon Syrup - Sweetly Light - www.sweetlylight.com

Wild Blueberry Concentrate - Tree of Life - www.kehe.com (distributor)

Weights & Measurements To Make Your Life Simpler

Volume Measurements

U.S.—Imperial--Metric

1/4 teaspoon--1 milliliters

1/2 teaspoon--2 milliliters

1 teaspoon--5 milliliters

1 tablespoon--15 milliliters

2 tablespoons--1 fluid ounces--30 milliliters

1/4 cup--2 fluid ounces--60 milliliters

1/3 cup--3 fluid ounces--80 milliliters

1/2 cup--4 fluid ounces--120 milliliters

2/3 cup--5 fluid ounces--160 milliliters

3/4 cup--6 fluid ounces--180 milliliters

1 cup--8 fluid ounces--240 milliliters

1 pint--16 fluid ounces

1 quart--32 fluid ounces

1 gallon--128 fluid ounces

Simplified

Dash--Less than 1/8 teaspoon

3 teaspoons--1 tablespoon

16 tablespoons--1 cup

1 cup--1/2 pint

2 cups--1 pint

2 pints--4 cups--1 quart

4 quarts--16 cups--1 gallon

8 quarts--1 peck

4 pecks--1 bushel

Tablespoons to Cups

4 tablespoons--1/4 cup

5 tablespoons plus 1 teaspoon--1/3 cup

8 tablespoons--1/2 cup

10 tablespoons plus 2 teaspoons--2/3 cup

12 tablespoons--3/4 cup

16 tablespoons--1 cup

Liters

Liters	Ounces	Approximate Realistic
1 Liter	33.814023	4 cups plus almost 1/4 cup
2 Liter	67.628046	8 1/4 cups plus 3 tablespoons
3 Liter	101.44207	12 1/2 cups plus almost 3 tablespoons

Length Measurements

U.S.--Metric

1/4 inch--6 centimeters

1/2 inch--1.25 centimeters

1 inch--2.5 centimeters

2 inches--5 centimeters

4 inches--11 centimeters

6 inches--15 centimeters

8 inches--20 centimeters

10 inches--25 centimeters

12 inches--30 centimeters

Pan Sizes

U.S.--Metric

8" cake pan--20 x 4 cm sandwich or cake pan

9" cake pan--23 x 3.5 cm sandwich or cake pan

11" x 7" baking pan--28 x 18 cm baking pan

15" x 10" baking pan--38 x 25.5 cm baking tin (Swiss roll pan)

1 1/2 qt baking dish--1.5 liter baking dish

2 qt baking dish--2 liter baking dish

2 qt rectangular baking dish--30 x 19 cm baking dish

9" pie pan--22 x 4 x 23 x 4 cm pie pan

7" or 8" springform pan--18 or 20 cm springform or loose-bottom cake pan

9" x 5" loaf pan--23 x 13 or 2 lb. narrow loaf tin or paté pan

Weight Measurements

U.S. Ounces	U.S. Pounds	Metric
1 ounce		30 grams
2 ounces		60 grams
4 ounces	1/4 pound	115 grams
5 ounces	1/3 pound	145 grams
6 ounces		170 grams
7 ounces		200 grams
8 ounces	1/2 pound	230 grams
10 ounces		285 grams
12 ounces	3/4 pound	340 grams
14 ounces		400 grams
16 ounces	1 pound	455 grams
35.2 ounces	2.2 pounds	1 kilogram

Temperatures

Fahrenheit—Centigrade

140°---60°	325°---163°
160°---71°	350°---177°
180°---82°	375°---191°
200°---93°	400°---204°
225°---107°	425°---218°
250°---121°	450°---232°
275°---135°	475°---246°
300°---149°	500°---260°

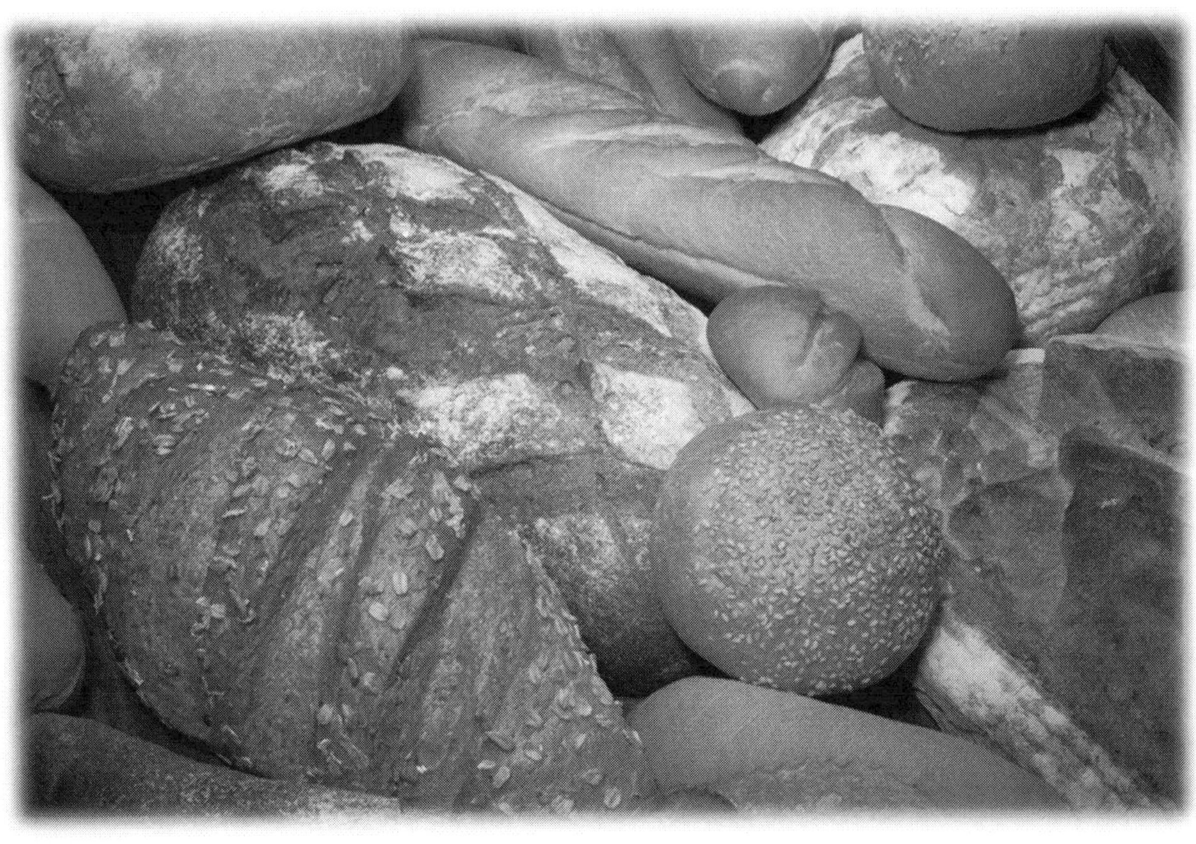

BREADS

When we first went gluten free, a truly satisfying bread always seemed to be out of reach. We tweaked recipes by substituting various flours for soy, sorghum, almond, barley, oat, rye, spelt, and chia. We eliminated milk, soy milk, almond milk, and buttermilk. We removed sugar, honey, fructose, Spenda® and every other conventional sweetener. Each recipe provided its own challenges regarding texture and taste, and these recipes represent the best of our efforts.

Since yeast and vinegar can be triggers for Candida, the majority of our recipes use baking powder and/or baking soda. However, we have included two recipes containing yeast and a small amount of vinegar.

Basic Pancakes

There are numerous recipes for gluten-free pancakes, which can be as simple or exotic as your imagination can take you. This recipe is basic yet delicious and easy to make. The original recipe was from the glutenfreeclub.com, a wonderful source of information with recipes for Celiacs and those who are gluten intolerant. We made some modifications to eliminate ingredients that caused Kris problems and invite you to add your own touches to create the taste you want. June

Makes: Approximately 16 pancakes
Prep Time: 15 minutes
Cook Time: 20 minutes

Ingredients:

1 cup rice flour
1/2 cup gram or bean flour
1/2 cup potato starch
1 tablespoon plus 1 teaspoon Baking Powder (see recipe in Mixes)
1 teaspoon baking soda
1 teaspoon salt

---

4 eggs, beaten
1 cup rice milk
2 tablespoons oil
2 tablespoons Frontier Non-Alcoholic Vanilla
1 tablespoon vegetable glycerine
8 drops SweetLeaf liquid stevia

Kitchen Tools:

Measuring cups and spoons
Handheld mixer or whisk
Medium and small mixing bowls
Griddle or large skillet

Instructions:

1. Measure the rice flour, gram (or bean) flour, potato starch, baking powder, baking soda, and salt in a medium bowl. Stir until well mixed.
2. Put eggs, rice milk, oil, vanilla, vegetable glycerine, and liquid stevia in a small bowl. Beat briefly with a whisk or mixer.
3. Pour liquids into dry mixture, and gently stir or mix on low just until combined. If there are a few small lumps in the batter, they will dissolve upon cooking. Do not over beat the batter.
4. Spray the griddle with oil and heat on medium to medium high heat. You'll know it's the right temperature when a drop of water skitters around like a preschooler on sugar.
5. Drop approximately 1/4 cup of batter on the hot skillet. When the tops bubble up, flip the pancakes over and cook for another minute or less. Remove to a warmed plate until all pancakes are made.
6. Serve hot with your favorite buttery spread and tapioca syrup, Sweet Berry Sauce or Caramel Syrup (see recipes in Sauces).

Variations:

Blueberry Pancakes: Add 1/2 cup fresh washed blueberries to batter just before cooking.

Cinnamon Pancakes: Add 1 teaspoon ground cinnamon to the flour mixture and increase liquid stevia to 10 drops.

Sweet Potato Flour Pancakes

I was tired of the same old taste for breakfast, which prompted me to think outside the box for a new pancake recipe. We are always trying to incorporate more vegetables into our diet and I had sweet potato flour, aka camote flour, in the cupboard. The challenge was to design a new taste and once again, our kitchen turned into a food lab. With a little bit of tweaking, we produced a flavorful pancake with gentle, sweet potato overtones that goes perfectly with bacon. Kris

Makes: 30 4" pancakes
Prep Time: 25 minutes
Cook Time: 20 minutes

Ingredients:

1/2 cup rice flour
1 cup sweet potato (camote) flour
1/2 cup potato starch
1 tablespoon plus 1 teaspoon Baking Powder (see recipe in Mixes)
1 teaspoon baking soda
1 teaspoon salt
1/2 teaspoon nutmeg

---

4 eggs, beaten
2 tablespoons canola oil
2 tablespoons Frontier Non-Alcoholic Vanilla
1 tablespoon brown rice syrup
12 drops SweetLeaf English Toffee liquid stevia

---

1 cup rice milk

Kitchen Tools:

Measuring cups and spoons

Handheld mixer

Medium and small mixing bowls

Griddle or large skillet

Instructions:

1. Measure the rice flour, sweet potato flour, potato starch, baking powder, baking soda, salt, and nutmeg in a medium bowl. Stir until well mixed.
2. Put eggs, oil, vanilla, brown rice syrup, and liquid stevia in a small bowl. Beat briefly with the electric mixer. Add the rice milk and mix well.
3. Pour liquids into dry mixture and beat for 30 seconds until smooth.
4. Spray the griddle with oil and heat on medium high heat until a drop of water will bounce around. When griddle is hot, reduce heat to medium.
5. Drop large spoons of batter on the hot skillet. When the tops bubble up a bit, flip pancakes over and cook for another minute or less. Watch carefully as they will brown quickly.
6. Serve hot with your favorite buttery spread, agave, tapioca syrup, or coconut nectar.

Variations:

Sautéed Apple Topping: If you can tolerate apples, peel, core, and slice apples. Sauté in buttery spread with a little cinnamon until barely soft. Add a bit of your preferred sweetener, if desired, and serve over pancakes.

Belgian Waffles

Belgian Waffles became popular during the 1964 New York World's Fair and were introduced by Maurice Vermersch of Brussels, Belgium. Originally called Brussels Waffles, Vermersch changed the name when he realized how geographically challenged Americans were. His waffles were served with whipped cream and strawberries and sold for $1. The cost today would be $7 at the rate of inflation. (Belgian Waffle)

The deeper "pockets" of Belgian waffles differentiate them from standard waffles. The crispy outside and soft inside is their trademark, and this recipe will give you this same texture. The stiffened egg whites folded into the batter give them lightness. This recipe was adapted from one found on glutenfreeclub.com, a comprehensive site with oodles of recipes and information about living successfully with Celiac Disease. Kris

Makes: 20 4" x 4" waffles

Prep Time: 30 minutes

Cook Time: 20 minutes (times vary according to your waffle iron)

Ingredients:

4 egg whites (retain yolks)

---

1 1/2 cups rice flour

1 cup potato starch

1/2 cup gram or bean flour

2 tablespoons Baking Powder (see recipe in Mixes)

1 teaspoon salt

---

4 egg yolks

1/4 cup canola oil

1 tablespoon vegetable glycerine

---

2 cups rice milk

2 tablespoons Frontier Non-Alcoholic Vanilla

Kitchen Tools:

Handheld mixer

Large bowl

Medium mixer bowl

Small bowl

Measuring cups and spoons

Rubber spatula (preferably large)

Belgian waffle maker

Instructions:

1. Using a handheld mixer in a medium mixer bowl, beat egg whites on low for 1 to 2 minutes. This will produce small bubbles as a base. Increase speed to high and beat until stiff peaks form. Set aside.
2. In a large bowl, stir together rice flour, potato starch, gram or bean flour, baking powder, and salt. If flours are lumpy, use a wire whisk to gently smooth out and incorporate the dry ingredients.
3. In a separate small bowl and using a handheld mixer, beat the egg yolks, oil, and vegetable glycerine. Add rice milk and vanilla and combine well.
4. Add egg yolk mixture to flours and beat until smooth.
5. Gently fold the egg whites into the batter with a large rubber spatula until the two are combined. Batter should have 1/2" bits of stiffened egg whites visible but resist the urge to make it smooth.
6. Heat waffle maker and, if necessary, brush with stir-fry tea oil or other high-heat oil to keep waffles from sticking. Follow the manufacturer's instructions for your waffle maker to achieve perfect waffles.
7. Serve warm with buttery spread and agave (if tolerated), plain tapioca syrup, Sweet Berry Sauce, Caramel Syrup (see recipes in Sauces), or other low-glycemic topping of your choice.

Works Cited

Belgian Waffle. Web. Published April 27, 2010 at 10:16 PM. Retrieved February 2, 2013 2013, from http://www.belgianwaffle.org/belgian-waffle/

Incredible Crepes

The inspiration for this recipe came from several recipes, like French Crepes from the Food Allergy Cookbook by Lucinda Bruce-Gardyne, published by The Reader's Digest, and French Pancakes from Betty Crocker's New Picture Cookbook, published by McGraw Hill Book Company, circa 1961. We added and tweaked ingredients until we got the exact results we wanted.

If you've never made crepes, you'll find them easy to mix up and cook. The key is to use a nonstick 6" skillet. The results are deliciously elegant, lending themselves to either savory or sweet fillings. June

Makes: 20 crepes
Prep Time: 15 minutes
Cook Time: 1 hour

Ingredients:

1 cup white rice flour
1/2 cup brown rice flour
1/2 cup tapioca flour
1/2 cup arrowroot starch
2 teaspoons salt
1 teaspoon Baking Powder (see recipe in Mixes)

---

4 eggs
3 cups rice milk
3 tablespoons grapeseed oil
8 drops SweetLeaf liquid stevia

Additional oil for pan

Kitchen Tools:

Whisk or handheld mixer

2 medium mixing bowls

Measuring spoons and cups

1 or 2 6" nonstick skillets

A flexible nylon spatula for flipping crepes

Instructions:

1. Thoroughly mix together the rice flours, tapioca flour, arrowroot starch, salt, and baking powder.
2. In a separate bowl, beat the eggs and add the rice milk, grapeseed oil, and stevia.
3. Pour dry ingredients into the liquid and mix well. Batter will be very thin.
4. Heat skillets over medium heat with a tiny bit of oil until oil is hot but not smoking. Pour off excess oil.
5. Stir the batter occasionally, as the flours will settle. Pour a scant 1/4 cup of batter into the skillet. Tip and turn the skillet until the bottom is evenly coated. When crepe begins to show a bit of brown around the edges in 1 to 2 minutes, gently ease spatula under the crepe and flip it over. Cook for an addition 30 seconds to 1 minute.
6. Remove to a plate and continue until all crepes have been made. They will keep for 4 days, if refrigerated.

Tip: Leftover crepes can be filled with ice cream and drizzled with a sauce for a delicious dessert.

Cream Puffs

Cream puffs are a versatile and creative way to present any type of filling—from your favorite ice cream to a savory filling. My first attempt at this recipe the way it came off the internet had me in giggles as I picked bits of dough out of my hair and off the ceiling. I believe cooking should be fun and as Kris says, "If you're not making a mess, you're not having fun." I worked on those parts of the recipe that caused me so much fun and the results were extraordinary. June

Serves: 6
Prep Time: 30 minutes
Bake Time: 40 minutes

Ingredients:

1 cup water
1/2 cup shortening
1/2 teaspoon salt
5 drops SweetLeaf liquid stevia

2/3 cup rice flour
1/3 cup potato starch

---

4 eggs

Kitchen Tools:

2-quart saucepan
Measuring cups and spoons
Your favorite stirring spoon
Stand mixer (not portable)
Parchment paper

Instructions:

1. Preheat oven to 450 degrees F (232 degrees C). Line a large baking sheet with parchment paper and set aside.
2. Combine water, shortening, salt, and stevia in a medium saucepan. Bring to a rapid boil.
3. Mix flours together and add to water and shortening. Stir vigorously until mixture forms a ball and leaves the sides of the pan.
4. Remove from heat and cool slightly.
5. Put mixture in a large, deep mixer bowl and beat for 1 minute. Add one egg at a time, while beating on as high a level as possible without having to dodge flying dough. Don't worry if dough isn't smooth. After adding the 4th egg, it will be fine.
6. Drop by tablespoons onto prepared baking sheet, forming 6 large cream puffs or 12 smaller ones, depending on your ultimate goal. Leave enough room for cream puffs to expand.
7. Bake for 20 minutes, then reduce heat to 350 degrees (177 degrees C). Bake for an additional 20 minutes.
8. Remove from oven and, if you are not using the puffs immediately, prick with a knife to let steam escape.
9. Cut off tops and stuff with your favorite filling.

Burger Buns aka Mousetrack Biscuits

It is a struggle to find satisfying recipes for breads and buns that do not have yeast, and the slightly sweet, spongy hamburger buns are something we really missed. Somehow, a hamburger just doesn't seem complete unless it's between a bun. We were fortunate to find this recipe for Burger Buns at glutenfreeclub.com, an excellent website put together by Angie Halten. She is dedicated to the dissemination of information on how to live gluten free and surrounds herself with professionals to share the most accurate facts.

Angie's recipe was called simply Burger Buns and called for sesame seeds to be sprinkled on top. The first time we tried this recipe, we only had black sesame seeds, which sent both Kris and me into giggles as we dubbed our creation Mousetrack Biscuits. We swapped out vegetable glycerine and liquid stevia for the sugar, rice milk for milk, and increased the salt slightly.

These buns are soft, spongy, and meet our criteria for tasty burger buns. We mix up the dry ingredients in batches and store in labeled plastic bags in the pantry for those nights when we have little time. We think you'll be as thrilled with the results as we are. June

Makes: 4 burger buns or 8 dinner rolls
Prep Time: 15 minutes
Bake Time: 15 minutes

Ingredients:

1/2 cup rice flour
1/2 cup potato starch
1/2 cup tapioca flour
2 teaspoons Baking Powder (see recipe in Mixes)
1 1/2 teaspoons xanthan gum
3/4 teaspoon salt

---

2 eggs
1/2 cup rice milk
1/3 cup oil
1 tablespoon vegetable glycerine
1/4 teaspoon SweetLeaf liquid stevia

Sesame seeds

Kitchen Tools:

Stand mixer
Rubber scraper
Measuring cups and spoons
Nonstick baking sheet

Instructions:

1. Preheat oven to 400 degrees F (204 degrees C). Oil baking sheet and set aside or cover baking sheet with parchment paper.
2. In mixer bowl, combine rice flour, potato starch, tapioca flour, baking powder, xanthan gum, and salt.
3. Add eggs, rice milk, oil, vegetable glycerine, and liquid stevia. Be prepared to carefully place your rubber scraper at the top of the mixer blades to keep the dough from "climbing" into the mechanism, and beat mixture until well combined, smooth, and glossy.
4. Drop two or three tablespoons of dough onto the baking sheet to make each of the 4 buns. Try to keep them uniform in shape and size. Allow enough room for the buns to expand.
5. Sprinkle the tops with sesame seeds and bake for 15 minutes or until lightly browned, but do not under bake. If you are making several dinner rolls instead, reduce baking time by 5 minutes and test for doneness.
6. Remove from oven and transfer to a plate. Cover with a clean cloth to keep warm. Use within 2 days. As with many gluten free breads, these buns begin to taste dry after 48 hours.

Variations:

Hot Dog Rolls: Put dough in a plastic bag, cut a corner of the bag to form a pastry bag, and form into 4" long rolls. Adjust baking time as needed.

Onion Rolls: Mix 3 tablespoons dried minced onion into liquids. Bake as directed.

Dinner Rolls: Use standard muffin pan and oil 8 muffin papers. Divide dough evenly among the muffin papers and bake for 15 minutes.

Onion Dill Dinner Rolls: Add 1 teaspoon Mrs. Dash Onion & Herb mix and 2 teaspoons dried dill weed. Use standard muffin pan and oil 8 muffin papers. Divide dough evenly among the muffin papers and bake for 15 minutes.

Tip: Leftover buns make a great breakfast sandwich with egg and bacon or sausage. Any buns left over after 2 days can be made into bread crumbs and frozen for future use.

English Muffins

Kris was lamenting the fact that English muffins contain yeast and other ingredients she could not have. She had pretty much given up on breads in general except for the recipes we had developed, but she still yearned for toasted English muffins and jam. When I searched the Internet for possibilities, I found a recipe at www.thedailydietribe.com, a website with recipes and great information on gluten free baking. We swapped out quinoa flour, 5 Flour Mix, potato flour, and oat flour for almond flour; cream of buckwheat cereal for Bob's Red Mill Mighty Tasty Hot Cereal; added a bit of sweetener, and increased the salt. This easy recipe has no eggs and requires no mixer.

We were thrilled with the hearty, whole-grain taste and think you will like it too. After cooling thoroughly, keep muffins stored in an airtight container or slice and freeze for future use. June

Makes: 8 English Muffins
Prep Time: 20 minutes
Rest Time: 10 minutes
Bake Time: 40 minutes

Ingredients:

1 cup oat flour
3/4 cup potato starch
1/2 cup Five Flour Mix (see recipe in Mixes)
1/4 cup quinoa flour
1/4 cup potato flour
3 tablespoons plus 1 teaspoon dry cream of buckwheat cereal
3 tablespoons chopped sunflower seeds
1 tablespoon plus 1 teaspoon Baking Powder (see recipe in Mixes)
2 1/2 teaspoons xanthan gum or guar gum
2 teaspoons sea salt

---

1 1/2 cups water
2 tablespoons ground flax seed

1/4 cup oil
1 tablespoon vegetable glycerine
1/4 teaspoon SweetLeaf liquid stevia

Kitchen Tools:

Medium bowl

Small bowl

Rubber scraper

Measuring cups and spoons

Large baking sheet

Parchment paper

Instructions:

1. Preheat oven to 350 degrees F (177 degrees C). Cover baking sheet with parchment paper and set aside.
2. In a medium bowl, stir dry ingredients together and mix well.
3. Measure water and stir in ground flax seed. Let sit 5 minutes.
4. In a small bowl, stir together the oil, vegetable glycerine, and stevia. Add flax seed water mixture and mix well. Pour into dry ingredients, stirring until completely mixed. Let mixture rest for 10 minutes to improve texture.
5. Drop heaping 1/3 cups of dough onto parchment paper, keeping space in between muffins. Form into 8 flat muffins, no thicker than 3/4", reshaping as necessary to even out the round shape.
6. Bake for 50 minutes total, turning the pan in the oven 180 degrees halfway though baking time. Edges should be golden brown to ensure insides are cooked. Let cool a few minutes before cutting in half. Store in an airtight plastic bag or covered container as soon as muffins are cooled.

Note: English muffins will keep for 3 days or can be frozen when cooled. Slice before freezing.

Note: The outside is intentionally crusty, so if you prefer a softer muffin, microwave briefly to soften. Muffins toast well, and toasting will give you a different flavor and texture.

Cornbread

It was a Sunday late afternoon, and I had spent three hours at my son's baseball game. I needed some time to myself and dearly needed a creative "fix" I could only get in the kitchen. I thought that cornbread would be a perfect addition to our dinner that evening. The goal was to create an end product that was moist and less grainy than traditional cornbread but with more texture and character than a cake. The corn flour, as well as the chopped corn, made this recipe come together in a way that exceeded my expectations.

Serve with Tomato-less Chili (see recipe in Soups, Stews & Casseroles), for breakfast, or as an easy snack. Kris

Serves: 6

Prep Time: 30 minutes

Bake Time: 20 to 25 minutes

Ingredients:

1 cup frozen corn, thawed or canned corn, well drained

---

3 tablespoons hot water

1 tablespoon ground flax seed

---

1 1/2 cups rice milk

3 tablespoons Spectrum Butter Flavor Shortening, melted

2 tablespoons vegetable glycerine

1/2 teaspoon SweetLeaf Vanilla Creme liquid stevia

---

1 1/4 cups corn flour (masa)

1/4 cup rice flour

1 tablespoon Baking Powder (see recipe in Mixes)

1 teaspoon salt

Kitchen Tools:

Food processor

Stand mixer

Medium bowl

Measuring cups and spoons

Whisk

8" x 8" baking dish

Instructions:

1. Preheat oven to 450 degrees F (232 degrees C). Place baking dish in the oven and let it heat while making the batter.
2. Put corn in food processor and process briefly to chop into smaller pieces.
3. Mix ground flax seed in 3 tablespoons of hot water. Let stand 10 minutes.
4. Put rice milk, melted shortening, vegetable glycerine, and stevia in the mixer bowl. Beat until combined. Shortening may reconstitute but this will not affect the end product.
5. Measure corn flour, rice flour, baking powder, and salt into a medium bowl. Gently whisk to combine well.
6. Add dry ingredients, reserved chopped corn, and flax seed mixture to the mixer bowl. Beat just until combined.
7. Remove hot baking dish from oven and spray with oil (not olive oil, please). Smooth batter into hot pan and bake for 20 to 25 minutes until toothpick inserted into the center comes out clean. Serve warm or cold.

Orange Poppy Seed Bread

We were feeling creative and had a desire to combine new flavors in a bread. We consulted several cookbooks, brainstormed possibilities, and settled on the combination of orange and poppy seed. We were inspired by Gail Burton's Poppy Seed and Orange Loaf recipe in The Candida Control Cookbook, Third Edition, published by Aslan Press, copyright 1989, and used her recipe as a launch pad for the flavor and texture we wanted. When we substituted for the ingredients in Ms. Burton's recipe that caused us problems, much to our surprise, the end product was a total failure. Using our best knowledge of food science, we systematically added ingredients and flavors, adjusted measurements, and tossed out our failures. By the time we reached an Orange Poppy Seed Bread we could be proud of, it no longer resembled the original recipe but, instead, we had a new bread to add to our list of favorites. Our thanks to Ms. Burton for the inspiration she provided. June

Serves: 6
Prep Time: 35 minutes
Bake Time: 50 minutes

Ingredients:

2 large eggs

1/2 cup coconut milk
1/2 cup water
3 tablespoons vegetable glycerine
2 teaspoons SweetLeaf Valencia Orange liquid stevia
2 teaspoons Frontier orange flavoring
1 teaspoon cranberry concentrate

---

1 1/4 cups Five Flour Mix (see recipe in Mixes)
1 cup Bette Hagman's Feather light Flour Mix (see recipe in Mixes)
1/4 cup coconut flour
2 tablespoons buckwheat flour
2 teaspoons Baking Powder (see recipe in Mixes)
1 1/2 teaspoons ground nutmeg
1 1/8 teaspoons sea salt

1/4 cup shortening, melted

1/4 cup poppy seeds
2 tablespoons fresh orange zest

Kitchen Tools:

5" x 9" loaf pan

Aluminum foil

Mixer and medium bowl, plus stand or handheld mixer

Measuring cups and spoons

Box grater

Instructions:

1. Preheat oven to 350 degrees F (177 degrees C). To line the loaf pan with aluminum foil, cut a strip of foil long enough to cover bottom and sides plus a couple inches. Invert the loaf pan and form the foil over the bottom of the pan. Turn the pan right side up, place foil inside pan, and gently ease into corners and over the edges. Oil foil and set aside.
2. Wash orange, and using the fine side of a box grater, grate most of the orange peel. Measure out 2 lightly packed tablespoons of zest and set aside.
3. Break eggs into mixer bowl and beat on high for 1 minute.
4. Add coconut milk, water, vegetable glycerine, liquid stevia, orange flavoring, and cranberry concentrate. Beat on low to combine.
5. In a medium bowl, stir together Five Flour Mix, Featherlight Flour, coconut flour, buckwheat flour, baking powder, nutmeg, and salt. Add to mixer bowl and beat on low just until mixed.
6. Add melted shortening and mix for 2 minutes.
7. Fold poppy seeds and orange zest into batter. Pour into loaf pan and bake for 50 to 60 minutes. Loaf is done when a toothpick inserted in the center comes out clean. Cool on a rack before slicing.

Note: This recipe can be successfully "muffinized." Divide batter into 12 paper lined muffin pans, and bake at 350 degrees F (177 degrees C) for 25 to 30 minutes.

Zucchini Bread

Kris was given a beautiful, large, organic zucchini, just begging to be made into zucchini bread. The inspiration for this recipe was Kelly E. Keough's Zucchini Bread recipe in Sugar-Free Gluten-Free Baking and Desserts, copyright 2009, published by Ulysses Press. Since coconut oil can be a trigger for Candida, we substituted Spectrum shortening and grapeseed oil. We reworked the sweeteners and flavorings to give us a sweet, gentle bread with a hint of lemon flavoring.

You can easily change this recipe into Zucchini Muffins by simply baking in muffin pans for a shorter time. June

Makes: 1 loaf or 12 muffins
Prep Time: 40 minutes
Bake Time: 1 hour 10 minutes

Ingredients:

1 1/4 cups shredded fresh zucchini

---

1 tablespoon fresh grated lemon zest

---

1 1/2 cups Bette Hagman's Featherlight Flour Mix (see recipe in Mixes)
1/2 cup quinoa flakes
1 teaspoon baking soda
1 teaspoon Baking Powder (see recipe in Mixes)
1 teaspoon salt
1 teaspoon xanthan gum
1/2 teaspoon nutmeg
1/2 teaspoon Ginger-Free Pumpkin Pie Spice (see recipe in Mixes)

1/2 cup rice milk or hemp milk
1/4 cup ground flaxseeds

---

1 large egg
3 tablespoons vegetable glycerine
2 tablespoons grapeseed oil
2 tablespoons Spectrum shortening, melted
2 tablespoons Frontier Non-Alcoholic Vanilla
2 1/4 teaspoons SweetLeaf Vanilla Creme liquid stevia
1/4 teaspoon Frontier Alcohol Free Lemon Flavor

Kitchen Tools:

Mixer bowl and medium bowl
Measuring cups and spoons
Stand or handheld mixer
8" x 4" x 2" loaf pan
Cup or small bowl
Aluminum foil
Box grater

Instructions:

1. Preheat oven to 350 degrees F (177 degrees C). To line the loaf pan with aluminum foil, cut a strip of foil long enough to cover bottom and sides plus a couple inches. Invert the loaf pan and form the foil over the bottom of the pan. Turn the pan right side up, place foil inside pan, and gently ease into corners and over the edges. Oil the foil and set aside.
2. Wash zucchini and grate, using the side with the finer holes. Lightly pack into measuring cups and set aside.
3. Wash lemon and, using the fine side of the grater, make lemon zest. Measure out 1 tablespoon, loosely packed, and set aside.
4. In a medium bowl, combine flour mix, quinoa flakes, baking soda, baking powder, salt, xanthan gum, nutmeg, and pumpkin pie spice. Set aside.
5. In a cup or small bowl, stir flaxseeds into the rice milk or hemp milk. Set aside.
6. In mixer bowl, beat together egg, vegetable glycerine, grapeseed oil, shortening, vanilla, liquid stevia, and lemon flavoring. Add flax seed mixture and zucchini. Mix well.
7. Add dry mixture to wet ingredients and stir until well combined. Allow batter to rest for 10 minutes while flour and quinoa flakes absorb liquids.
8. Spread batter in pan and bake for 1 hour 10 to 15 minutes until toothpick inserted in center comes out clean. Cool in the pan on a wire rack for 10 minutes. Remove from pan and continue to cool on wire rack before cutting.

Variations:

Zucchini Muffins: Oil muffin papers and evenly distribute batter to make 12 muffins. Bake at 350 degrees F (177 degrees C) for 35 minutes. Muffin papers will cling to muffins until thoroughly cooled.

Sunflower Seed Zucchini Bread: In the final stage, stir 1/2 cup roasted sunflower seeds into batter and follow baking directions.

Tip: If you don't quite have enough zucchini after grating, peel and grate enough carrot to make 1 1/4 cups.

Five Flour Bread

This recipe was inspired by Bette Hagman's Basic Yeast-free Bean Bread in her innovative cookbook, The Gluten-free Gourmet Bakes Bread, copyright 1999, published by Henry Holt and Company, LLC. Her recipe posed some problems for us, so we had to substitute for sorghum flour, brown sugar, butter, honey, and buttermilk. Our first loaf had to be rebaked but eventually found new life through bread pudding. Our second and third attempts became bread crumbs. By the sixth try, we got it right. This recipe uses our Five Flour Mix, so, if you use another flour combination, you may have to make adjustments to the recipe and may not achieve the results you desire.

If you're not familiar with Vitamin C crystals, they can be found in most health food stores and act as a dough enhancer in this recipe.

This bread is high, moist, a pale yellow in color, slightly sweet, and slices well. Use it not only for sandwiches but French toast, Bread Pudding (see recipe in Desserts), or Ham and Cheese Strata (see recipe in Eggs). June

Makes: 1 loaf
Prep Time: 30 minutes
Bake Time: 1 hour 25 minutes

Ingredients:

3 3/4 cups Five Flour Mix (see recipe in Mixes)
1/4 cup coconut flour
1 tablespoon xanthan gum
1 tablespoon Baking Powder (see recipe in Mixes)
2 teaspoons Egg Replacer
1 1/2 teaspoons salt
1 teaspoon baking soda
1 teaspoon Vitamin C crystals

---

3 eggs plus 2 egg whites

1/4 cup plus 2 tablespoons buttery spread, melted
2 tablespoons vegetable glycerine
1/2 teaspoon SweetLeaf liquid stevia

---

1 1/2 cups rice milk
1 tablespoon cream of tartar

Kitchen Tools:

Loaf pan

Mixer bowl and medium bowl

Handheld mixer

Aluminum foil

Instructions:

1. Preheat oven to 325 degrees F (163 degrees C). Line loaf pan with aluminum foil and grease bottom and sides.
2. In a medium bowl, whisk together flour, coconut flour, xanthan gum, baking powder, egg replacer, salt, baking soda, and Vitamin C crystals. Set aside.
3. In a mixer bowl, beat the eggs and whites on high for 1 minute. Add melted buttery spread, vegetable glycerine, and liquid stevia. Beat briefly to combine.
4. Measure out rice milk and stir cream of tartar into milk until dissolved. Add to mixer bowl and beat briefly.
5. Add flour mixture to liquids and stir just until combined. Small lumps will disappear in the baking process.
6. Pour into prepared pan and bake uncovered for 30 minutes. Remove from oven and cover pan loosely with foil. Return to oven and bake for 55 minutes longer until bread is golden brown and pops back up when top is tapped.

Variations:

Five Flour Biscuits: Oil 16 muffin papers and divide batter evenly or use 12 muffin papers and a mini loaf pan. Bake at 325 degrees F (163 degrees C) for 40 minutes.

Focaccia Bread

Focaccia bread is one of life's great gastronomic delights and, until we searched out a recipe specifically without yeast, I didn't think it would be possible to make a focaccia bread with the taste and texture we were looking for. This recipe came off the Bob's Red Mill website and, with changes to suit our taste and dietary needs, it proved to be a new favorite in our house. Try it with quiche, soup, or your favorite main course for a wonderful addition to your meal. Kris

Serves: 8
Prep Time: 30 minutes
Bake Time: 30 to 35 minutes

Ingredients:

1 3/4 cups gluten free oat flour
1/2 cup plus 1/3 cup tapioca flour
2/3 cup potato starch
1 1/4 teaspoons baking soda
1 teaspoon Baking Powder (see recipe in Mixes)
1 teaspoon salt
3/4 teaspoon onion powder
1/2 teaspoon xanthan gum
1/2 teaspoon unflavored gelatin powder
1/2 teaspoon crushed rosemary

---

2 eggs
1 cup club soda
2 tablespoons olive oil
1 teaspoon vegetable glycerine
5 drops SweetLeaf liquid stevia

Topping Ingredients:

1 tablespoon olive oil

1/2 teaspoon Italian Herb Mix (see recipe in Mixes)
1/4 teaspoon salt

Kitchen Tools:

Stand mixer

Measuring cups and spoons

Rubber spatula

11" x 7" baking dish

Parchment paper

Instructions:

1. Preheat oven to 375 degrees F (191 degrees C). Cut parchment paper to fit in the bottom of the pan and set aside.
2. Measure dry ingredients into a large mixing bowl and stir to combine. Add eggs, club soda, oil, vegetable glycerine, and stevia. Using regular beaters as opposed to dough hooks, beat until smooth.
3. Spread evenly in pan. Brush top with olive oil and sprinkle with Italian Herb Mix and salt.
4. Bake for 30 to 35 minutes until top is well browned. Do not under bake. Slice into thick slices. Serve with your favorite buttery spread.

Three Seed Bread

The original inspiration for this recipe was from 125 Best Gluten-Free Recipes by Donna Washburn and Heather Butt, published by Robert Rose, entitled Country Harvest Loaf. We were thrilled to find multigrain-tasting bread that was not only delicious, but also had just the right texture. It was far superior to any other non-yeast bread we had tried, but when we developed allergies to some of the original ingredients, we had to improvise.

Changes to make it more allergy-friendly included eliminating the honey and substituting vegetable glycerine and liquid stevia, as well as swapping out rice milk for cow's milk. We also increased the salt for taste and removed the vinegar.

The moist texture and nutty flavor are a perfect accompaniment to a bowl of soup or a large salad. June

Makes: 1 loaf
Prep Time: 25 minutes
Rest Time Before Baking: 30 minutes
Bake Time: 1 hour 25 minutes

Ingredients:

1 2/3 cups plus 3 tablespoons rice milk
1/4 cup ground flaxseed

---

1 3/4 cups rice flour
1/2 cup cornstarch
1/2 cup tapioca flour
1/2 cup sunflower seeds
3 tablespoons sesame seeds
1 tablespoon plus 1 1/2 teaspoons Baking Powder (see recipe in Mixes)
2 teaspoons xanthan gum
1 3/4 teaspoons salt

1/4 cup vegetable oil
3 tablespoons vegetable glycerine
3/4 teaspoon SweetLeaf liquid stevia

Kitchen Tools:

9" x 5" loaf pan

2 small bowls

Large mixing bowl

Medium bowl

Stand or handheld mixer

Instructions:

1. Oil a 9" x 5" loaf pan or line pan with foil and oil. Set aside.
2. Measure rice milk and flaxseed into a small bowl. Stir to mix and refrigerate while you continue with the next steps.
3. In a mixer bowl, stir together the rice flour, cornstarch, tapioca flour, sunflower seeds, sesame seeds, baking powder, xanthan gum, and salt. Set aside.
4. In a separate small bowl, mix the vegetable oil, vegetable glycerine, and liquid stevia. Add the rice milk and flaxseed mixture. Mix well.
5. Add liquids to the dry ingredients in the mixer bowl and mix just until lumps no longer remain. Spread evenly in the pan and let rest for 30 minutes.
6. Meanwhile, preheat convection oven to 300 degrees F (149 degrees C). Bake for 1 hour and 25 minutes. The toothpick inserted in the center test does not work with this recipe, so do not under bake. Remove from oven, let cool in the pan for 10 minutes, remove from pan, and cool completely on a rack before cutting.

Tip: Leftover bread is sensational in Bread Pudding (see recipe in Desserts).

Sandwich Yeast Bread

If you battle Candida, unfortunately, you should stay away from yeast, sugar, and vinegar. If this is the case, this recipe isn't for you. But if Candida is not an issue, you'll find this bread tasty and great for sandwiches, bread pudding, and French toast. The loaf is pale yellow and holds together well. As with all fresh baked gluten-free breads, this bread is at its best in the first two days after baking. June

Makes: 1 loaf
Prep Time: 30 minutes
Rise Time: Approximately 30 to 45 minutes
Bake Time: 1 hour

Dry Ingredients:

1 1/4 cups white rice flour
1/2 cup millet flour
1/2 cup tapioca flour
1/2 cup potato starch
1/4 cup coconut flour
2 teaspoons xanthan gum
1 1/2 teaspoons salt
2 1/2 teaspoons active dry yeast

Wet Ingredients:

3 eggs

---

1 1/2 cups minus 2 tablespoons 110 degree F (43 degrees C) water
1/4 cup Spectrum palm oil shortening, melted
2 tablespoons vegetable glycerine
1 teaspoon apple cider vinegar
1/2 teaspoon SweetLeaf liquid stevia

Kitchen Tools:

Stand mixer
Medium bowl
Mixer bowl
Measuring cups and spoons
Loaf pan
Aluminum foil

Instructions:

1. Preheat convection oven to 300 degrees F (149 degrees C) when time is right. To line the loaf pan with aluminum foil, cut a piece of foil long enough to give you a couple extra inches to work with. Turn pan upside down and form the foil over the bottom and sides of the pan. Flip pan over and gently ease foil into corners of pan and over the edges. Oil foil and set aside.
2. In a medium bowl, measure all dry ingredients together. Stir to ensure flours are well mixed and that any clumps of flour are broken up.
3. In a microwaveable bowl or cup, heat water for 1 minute.
4. In the mixer bowl, beat eggs until broken down. Add water, melted shortening, vegetable glycerine, vinegar, and liquid stevia. Beat briefly.
5. If you have an awesome mixer, add the flour all at once. Beat on high for 3 minutes, scraping down sides as necessary. Dough will become thick very quickly. If your mixer is a standard variety, gradually add the flour mixture and then beat for 3 minutes.
6. Spread dough evenly in prepared loaf pan. Oil a piece of waxed paper and place loosely over bread pan. Let rise in a warm place until bread reaches the top of the pan or no more than 1/2 inch above the pan. Here are some ways to encourage bread to rise:
   - Place a towel over a heating pad turned to medium. Cover bread pan with oiled waxed paper and allow bread to rise.
   - Heat a shallow pan of water to boiling and place on the bottom oven rack in an oven that is not on. Place bread pan without the waxed paper on the top rack, allowing enough head room for dough to rise in a closed oven.
   - Heat oven to no more than 150 degrees F (65 degrees C). Turn off oven and let bread rise in the oven with the door closed.
   - Get creative and, depending on where you live, what time of year it is, and what car you drive, put the bread pan covered with waxed paper in the back window in the sun to rise.
7. Bake loaf for 1 hour and cool on a rack before cutting. Store in a plastic bag in the refrigerator.

Tip: The level of sweetness is slight, so if you're looking for sweeter bread, increase the vegetable glycerine by 1 tablespoon and the liquid stevia by 1/4 teaspoon.

Variations:

Sesame Seed Bread: Add 1/4 cup sesame seeds to the flour mixture.

Note: If you do not have a convection oven, bake at 325 degrees F (163 degrees C) for 1 hour. Turn the pan 180 degrees halfway through baking.

Quarter Loaf Yeast Bread

We've tried many gluten free, yeast based bread recipes in the past few years. Admittedly, all of them were better than the commercial gluten-free breads we purchased, but still lacked some or all the important elements that make a great bread: taste, texture, slice-ability, and moistness.

This bread recipe began with good intentions and a bread machine. After two years of massive tweaking, we had the taste right but the texture was like a brick, and no matter what I did, the best I could get was a porous brick. In desperation, I threw myself on the mercy of Maureen Burke of One Dish Cuisine and tapped into her vast knowledge. She suggested a couple minor changes to ingredients but mentioned the awesome bread they make at their restaurant is simply oven baked.

This recipe got its name because it took 25 attempts to reach an end product that was spongy soft, slightly sweet, tasty, and one that slices well for toast or sandwiches. The directions are for a convection oven, as the oven fan creates more even heat for baking. If you have a conventional oven, you may have to experiment with temperature, timing, and turning the loaf 180 degrees halfway through baking.

Please note that yeast and vinegar are triggers for Candida, but if that is not an issue for you, give this recipe a try. The smell of baking bread in the house is intoxicating, and you won't be disappointed in the results. June

Makes: 1 loaf
Prep Time: 25 minutes
Rise Time: Approximately 30 minutes
Bake Time: 1 hour 35 minutes

Dry Ingredients:
2 cups Bette Hagman's Featherlight Flour Mix (see recipe in Mixes)
1/4 cup coconut flour
1/4 cup gram or bean flour
1/4 cup rice flour
1 tablespoon active dry yeast
2 teaspoons xanthan gum
2 teaspoons salt

Wet Ingredients:

3/4 cup water

3/4 cup rice milk, hemp milk, or other non-dairy alternative

---

2 eggs

1/4 cup Spectrum palm oil shortening, melted

3 tablespoons vegetable glycerine

1 teaspoon apple cider vinegar

1/2 teaspoon SweetLeaf liquid stevia

Kitchen Tools:

Stand mixer

Large mixer bowl

Medium bowl

Measuring cups and spoons

Loaf pan

Aluminum foil

Instructions:

1. Preheat convection oven to 300 degrees F (149 degrees C) when the time is right. To line the loaf pan with aluminum foil, cut a piece of foil long enough to give you a couple extra inches to work with. Turn pan upside down and form the foil over the bottom and sides of the pan. Flip pan over and gently ease foil into corners of pan and over the edges. Oil foil and set aside.
2. In a medium bowl, measure all dry ingredients together. Stir well to ensure flours are well mixed and that any clumps are incorporated.
3. In a microwaveable bowl or cup, heat water and rice milk for 1 minute. Liquid should be 110 degrees F (43 degrees C) when combined with egg.
4. In the mixer bowl, beat eggs until broken down. Add the water and rice milk, melted shortening, vegetable glycerine, vinegar, and liquid stevia. Beat briefly.
5. If you have an awesome mixer, add the flour all at once. Beat on high for 3 minutes, scraping down sides as necessary. If your mixer is a standard variety, gradually add the flour mixture and then beat for 3 minutes.
6. Spread dough evenly in loaf pan. Oil a piece of waxed paper and place loosely over bread pan. Let rise in a warm place until bread expands to top of pan. For ways to encourage bread to rise, see recipe for Sandwich Yeast Bread.

7. Bake loaf in convection oven at 300 degrees F (149 degrees C) for 1 hour 35 minutes. Cool on a rack before cutting and store in a plastic bag in the refrigerator.

Variations:

Sesame Seed: Add 1/4 cup sesame seeds to the flour mixture.

Buckwheat Bread: For a more whole wheat flavor, replace up to 2 tablespoons of bean flour with buckwheat flour and reduce liquid by 2 tablespoons. Buckwheat is gluten free—not actually wheat but related to rhubarb.

Note: If you do not have a convection oven, try baking at 325 degrees F (163 degrees C) for 1 hour 35 minutes. Turn the pan 180 degrees halfway through baking to encourage uniform browning.

MUFFINS

While muffins are technically a bread, we have given them their own section because of their portability and versatility. Muffins can be a take-along meal or a treat in a plain paper wrapper. We have combined our favorite flavors into delicious sweetness and tantalizing textures that will offer you variety in taste.

Almost any sweet bread recipe can be turned into muffins, so be sure to search out the Breads section for other recipes to "muffinize."

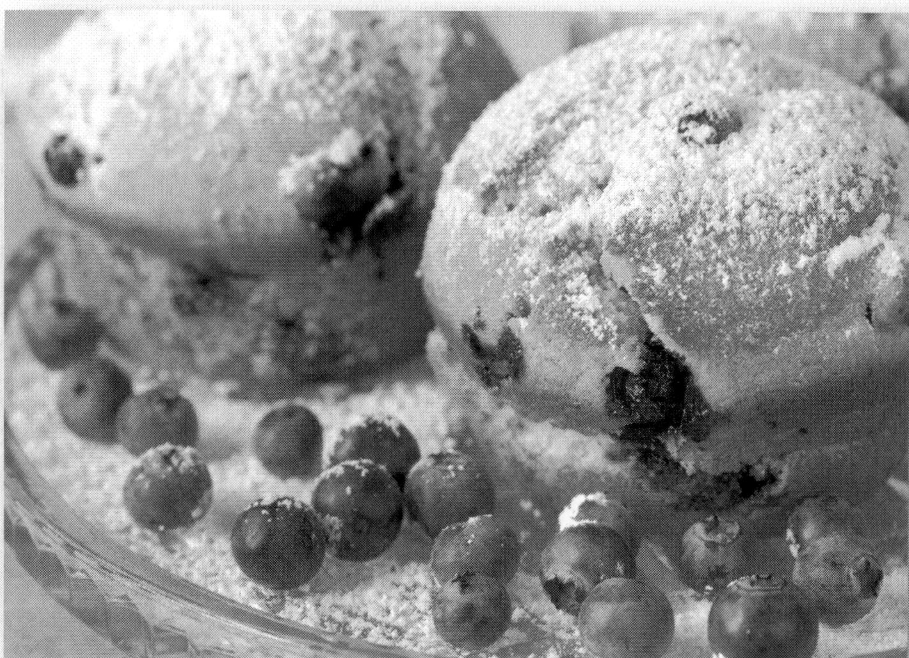

Blueberry Muffins

I must admit that, until I tried this recipe, I didn't think I liked blueberry muffins, or perhaps it was just all the chemicals and artificial flavors that went into commercial muffins to which my body objected. I was pleasantly surprised with my first bite, and these have become one of my favorite foods.

We took elements from our Carrot Muffin recipe and kept reworking the ingredients until we got the taste and texture we wanted. The end result is a muffin that is light, refreshing, and satisfyingly sweet. Fresh blueberries really work best, but if you must use frozen, thaw and drain them well, and you will still be pleased with the results. June

Makes: 12 muffins
Prep Time: 50 minutes
Bake Time: 25 to 30 minutes

Ingredients:

2 tablespoons lemon zest

---

2 1/4 cups Bette Hagman's Featherlight Flour Mix (see recipe in Mixes)
2 tablespoons quinoa flour
1 1/2 teaspoons xanthan gum
1 teaspoon baking soda
3/4 teaspoon salt
1/2 teaspoon Baking Powder (see recipe in Mixes)

---

2 eggs, beaten
3/4 cup seltzer water
3 tablespoons vegetable glycerine
2 tablespoons blueberry concentrate
1 3/4 teaspoons SweetLeaf Lemon Drop liquid stevia
1/2 teaspoon SweetLeaf Berry liquid stevia

1/4 cup coconut oil melted

---

2 cups frozen blueberries, thawed and well drained

---

2 tablespoons coconut sugar

Kitchen Tools:

Medium and small sized mixing bowls

Whisk or handheld electric mixer

Your favorite mixing spoon

Measuring cups and spoons

Muffin pan

Instructions:

1. Preheat oven to 350 degrees F (177 degrees C). Oil muffin pan and set aside. Do not use paper liners, as muffins will stick to the papers, even when cooled.
2. Wash lemon and using a fine side of grater, make 2 tablespoons of lemon zest. Set aside.
3. In a medium bowl, stir together flour mix, quinoa flour, xanthan gum, baking soda, salt, and baking powder.
4. Using the handheld mixer or a whisk in a small bowl, break down eggs. Thoroughly mix in the seltzer water, vegetable glycerine, blueberry concentrate, and liquid stevias.
5. Pour into dry mixture, add melted coconut oil, and beat until smooth. Mixture will become thick. Gently stir in lemon zest and blueberries.
6. Evenly fill muffin pan and sprinkle 1/2 teaspoon coconut sugar over each muffin. Bake for 30 to 35 minutes, until a toothpick inserted in the center comes out clean.
7. Transfer to a cooling rack and store muffins in a closed container when thoroughly cooled.

Carrot Muffins

Carrots are extremely versatile, and whoever thought to put them in cakes and muffins was an absolute genius. We like these soft muffins as they are, without frosting, but you can be the judge. Who would guess that something sweet could actually be good for you?

For an extra bit of sweetness and contrast, drizzle a bit of Caramel Syrup (see recipe in Sauces) over baked muffins. Kris

Makes: 12 muffins

Prep Time: 45 minutes

Bake Time: 20 to 25 minutes

Ingredients:

1/2 cup roasted sunflower seeds, chopped (optional)

---

2 cups shredded carrots

---

2 eggs
1/2 cup oil
1/4 cup vegetable glycerine
2 tablespoons Frontier Non-Alcoholic Vanilla
2 teaspoons SweetLeaf Apricot Nectar liquid stevia

---

1 1/2 cups Bette Hagman's Featherlight Flour Mix (see recipe in Mixes)
1 1/2 teaspoons xanthan gum
1 1/2 teaspoons cinnamon
1 teaspoon Ginger-Free Pumpkin Pie Spice (see recipe in Mixes)
1 teaspoon salt
1 teaspoon baking soda
1/2 teaspoon Baking Powder (see recipe in Mixes)
1/4 teaspoon ground cloves

---

1 tablespoon fresh orange zest or 1 teaspoon dried

Kitchen Tools:

Muffin pan and muffin papers

Mixer bowl

Small bowl

Stand mixer

Measuring cups and spoons

Food processor

Box grater

Instructions:

1. Preheat oven to 350 degrees F (177 degrees C). Place oiled muffin papers in pan and set aside.
2. Measure sunflower seeds into food processor and process briefly until seeds are chopped but not pulverized. Set aside.
3. Peel the carrots and either use a food processor or a box grater to coarsely grate. Set aside.
4. Break eggs into a mixer bowl and add the oil, vegetable glycerine, vanilla, and liquid stevia. Using a stand mixer, beat for 1 minute.
5. In the small bowl, stir together the flour, xanthan gum, cinnamon, pumpkin pie spice, salt, baking soda, baking powder, and ground cloves. Add to the liquid mixture and beat until mixture is smooth and thick. It will thicken very quickly, so, if necessary, use dough hooks or be prepared to place the flat part of the your rubber spatula gently above the beaters to discourage the dough from "climbing" into your mixer motor.
6. Wash a fresh orange. Using the small side of a box grater, grate orange zest and add to batter.
7. Stir in the sunflower seeds and carrots. Batter will be fairly stiff. Divide the batter evenly among the muffin papers and bake for 20 to 25 minutes until a toothpick in the center comes out clean, or a light touch in the center of a muffin springs back. Cool on a rack and store muffins in a closed container.

Variations:

Coconut Option: Stir 1/2 cup unsweetened shredded coconut into the batter with the sunflower seeds and carrots.

Chocolate Muffins

The inspiration for this recipe came from Flying Apron's Gluten-Free & Vegan Baking Book by Jennifer Katzinger, published by Sasquatch Books. Her dark chocolate muffins were simply superb but contained ingredients we needed to eliminate from our diet. To get just the taste and texture we wanted, we combined a number of flours with quinoa flakes. There are no eggs in this recipe, and you will not miss them. This rich, chocolate treat is enhanced when frosted with Choco-Coco-Berry Frosting (see recipe in Sauces) and perfect with a cup of coffee or your favorite tea. Kris

Makes: 9 muffins
Prep Time: 30 minutes
Rest Time: 10 minutes
Bake Time: 20 to 25 minutes

Ingredients:

1/4 cup plus 2 tablespoons brown rice flour
1/4 cup plus 2 tablespoons cocoa powder
1/4 cup white rice flour
1/4 cup quinoa flakes
2 tablespoons coconut flour
2 tablespoons bean flour
2 tablespoons chestnut flour
1 tablespoon dark cocoa powder
1 1/4 teaspoons baking soda
3/4 teaspoon sea salt

1/2 cup plus 2 tablespoons, plus 2 teaspoons water
1/3 cup canola oil
1/4 cup coconut milk
3 tablespoons vegetable glycerine
1 tablespoon Frontier Non-Alcoholic Vanilla
1 teaspoon SweetLeaf Chocolate Raspberry liquid stevia
1 teaspoon SweetLeaf English Toffee liquid stevia

Kitchen Tools:

Muffin pan

Muffin papers

Medium bowl

Whisk

Handheld or stand mixer

Instructions:

1. Preheat oven to 350 degrees F (177 degrees C). Place 9 greased muffin papers in the muffin pan and set aside.
2. In a medium bowl, whisk together the brown rice flour, cocoa powder, white rice flour, quinoa flakes, coconut flour, bean flour, chestnut flour, dark cocoa powder, baking soda, and salt. Set aside.
3. In mixer bowl, combine water, oil, coconut milk, vegetable glycerine, vanilla, and liquid stevias. Add the flour mixture and beat on high for 1 minute. Let batter rest for 10 minutes for quinoa flakes to absorb liquids.
4. Fill muffin papers and bake for 20 to 25 minutes or until a toothpick inserted into the muffin comes out clean. Remove muffins from pan and cool on a rack. Frost with Choco-Coco-Berry Frosting (see recipe in Sauces) when cooled, or enjoy plain.

Note: If baking less than a dozen muffins, preserve muffin pan by filling any empty cavity with water before baking.

Sweet Potato Muffins

We frequently buy a new product when we first see it and then figure out what to do with it later. I came home with sweet potato flour, otherwise known as camote flour, and was surprised when I Googled sweet potato flour for recipes, that there just weren't many recipes to be found.

It seemed pretty natural to combine this new flour with sweet potatoes, and the muffin format proved to be a good choice. We've combined sweet potato flour with a gluten-free flour blend to produce a sweet, soft, crunchy, healthy muffin. These muffins pack well in lunch boxes, and we think you'll love what you've created. Kris

Makes: 10 muffins
Prep Time: 35 minutes
Bake Time: 20 to 25 minutes

Ingredients:

3/4 cup Bette Hagman's Modified GF Flour Mix (see recipe in Mixes)
1/2 cup sunflower seeds or raw hemp seeds (optional)
1/4 cup sweet potato flour
2 teaspoons ground cinnamon
1 1/2 teaspoons Baking Powder (see recipe in Mixes)
1 teaspoon salt
1/2 teaspoon baking soda
1/2 teaspoon xanthan gum
1/4 teaspoon ground nutmeg
1/8 teaspoon ground cloves

---

1 egg
3/4 cup mashed sweet potatoes, fresh or canned
1/4 cup rice milk or hemp milk
1/4 cup canola oil
3 tablespoons vegetable glycerine
1 tablespoon Frontier Non-Alcoholic Vanilla
1 teaspoon SweetLeaf Apricot Nectar liquid stevia

Kitchen Tools:

Medium bowl

Slightly smaller bowl

Handheld mixer or whisk

Measuring cups and spoons

Muffin pan and papers

Instructions:

1. Preheat oven to 350 degrees F (177 degrees C). Place 10 oiled paper liners in the muffin pan. You can either spread a little oil around each paper or spray each one with a bit of oil.
2. Combine the flour mix, sunflower seeds, sweet potato flour, cinnamon, baking powder, salt, baking soda, xanthan gum, nutmeg, and cloves in a medium bowl. Stir well.
3. In a smaller bowl, combine the egg, sweet potatoes, rice milk, oil, vegetable glycerine, vanilla, and liquid stevia. Either whisk until well mixed, or use a handheld mixer.
4. Add wet ingredients to the flour mixture and stir until combined so there is no dry flour. Mixture will be quite stiff.
5. Evenly distribute batter among the muffin papers. Bake for 20 to 25 minutes until a toothpick inserted into the middle of a muffin comes out clean. Cool completely on a rack to encourage the papers not to stick to the muffin.

Note: After a day or so, the sunflower seeds will turn a pretty, bright green. This appears to be a chemical action between the seed's chlorogenic acid and the baking soda and baking powder. We experimented with reducing the quantities of the baking soda and baking powder but decided we'd rather have colorful seeds and a better texture.

Variations:

Coconut Option: Add 1/2 cup unsweetened coconut flakes in step 2, or replace sunflower seeds with coconut.

Hemp Hearts Option: Add 1/2 cup hemp seed hearts in step 2, or replace sunflower seeds.

French Puffs

The inspiration for these mini muffins was a recipe from A View With A Room, an exquisitely decorated Bed and Breakfast with a view of Mount Rainier in Puyallup, Washington. Check out the website at www.aviewwitharoom.net. Lenny Zimmerman is a natural at creative interior decorating who delights her guests with little visual treasures found in unlikely places. She has fabulous people skills that have her guests coming back year after year from all over the world.

To make this recipe allergy friendly, we replaced the sugar with flavored stevias, vegetable glycerine, and coconut sugar. We swapped out buttery spread for real butter, used gluten-free flour, and added xanthan gum.

These mini muffins are best served fresh out of the oven, still warm. The sweet buttery top is a perfect accompaniment to the slightly sweet muffin base. June

Makes: 18 mini muffins
Prep Time: 25 minutes
Bake Time: 15 to 20 minutes

Ingredients:

1 1/2 cups Bette Hagman's Modified GF Flour Mix (see recipe in Mixes)
1 1/2 teaspoons Baking Powder (see recipe in Mixes)
1/2 teaspoon salt
1/2 teaspoon xanthan gum
1/2 teaspoon ground nutmeg

---

1 large egg
1/2 cup coconut milk
1/3 cup melted buttery spread
3 tablespoons vegetable glycerine
3/4 teaspoon SweetLeaf Vanilla Creme liquid stevia
1/2 teaspoon SweetLeaf Orange liquid stevia

Glaze:

1/4 cup melted buttery spread

1/3 cup coconut sugar

1 teaspoon ground cinnamon

Kitchen Tools:

Medium bowl

2 small bowls

Measuring cups and spoons

Mini muffin pans and papers

Instructions:

1. Preheat oven to 350 degrees F (177 degrees C). Place 18 oiled mini muffin paper liners in the pans. You can either spread a little oil around each paper or spray each one with a bit of oil.
2. Combine the flour, baking powder, salt, xanthan gum, and nutmeg in a medium bowl. Blend well.
3. In a separate bowl, beat together the egg, coconut milk, buttery spread, vegetable glycerine, and liquid stevias.
4. Pour liquid into the flour mixture. Stir to blend, but do not over mix.
5. Fill prepared muffin papers evenly with the batter and bake for 15 to 20 minutes or until a toothpick inserted into the center comes out clean.
6. Melt buttery spread in a small bowl and set aside. Mix coconut sugar and cinnamon in a separate small bowl and set aside. While puffs are still warm, dip each one in melted buttery spread and then in coconut sugar. Serve immediately.

Veggie Biscuits

Bette Hagman's recipe for Vegetable Garden Muffins in her excellent cookbook, The Gluten-Free Gourmet Cooks Fast and Healthy, copyright 1996, published by Henry Holt and Company, LLC was the inspiration for these biscuits. This recipe is a great way to incorporate vegetables into baked goods. We were unsure whether to put this in the bread section or classify it as a muffin so, after a family vote, we opted to include it here to remind us that muffins don't have to be sweet to be satisfying.

The end product is slightly salty, sumptuous, and perfect served with a buttery spread. It's great for breakfast or with chili, soup, salad, or as an un-sweet snack. Kris

Makes: 12 biscuits
Prep Time: 40 minutes
Bake Time: 18 to 23 minutes

Ingredients:
2 cups Bette Hagman's Featherlight Flour Mix (see recipe in Mixes)
1 tablespoon plus 1 teaspoon Baking Powder (see recipe in Mixes)
2 teaspoons salt-free seasoning
1 1/2 teaspoons Egg Replacer
1 teaspoon baking soda
1 teaspoon Seasoned Salt (see recipe in Mixes)
1/2 teaspoon xanthan gum

---

2 eggs
3/4 cup coconut cream, at least 17% fat per 1/2 cup
1/4 cup rice milk
2 tablespoons vegetable oil
1 tablespoon vegetable glycerine

1/2 cup finely chopped or grated carrots
1/4 cup sweet onions, finely chopped
3 tablespoons chopped fresh parsley

Kitchen Tools:

Muffin pan and papers

Measuring cups and spoons

Mixing bowl

Handheld mixer

Box grater

Small bowl

Cutting board and your favorite chopping knife

Instructions:

1. Preheat oven to 400 degrees F (204 degrees C). Place greased muffin papers in muffin pan and set aside.
2. In a medium bowl, combine flour mix, baking powder, salt-free seasoning, egg replacer, baking soda, seasoned salt, and xanthan gum. Stir to mix and set aside.
3. In a small bowl, beat together the eggs, coconut cream, rice milk, oil, and vegetable glycerine. Stir in the carrots, onions, and parsley.
4. Add wet ingredients to dry ingredients. Stir just until mixture is moistened and no pockets of flour mixture remain.
5. Fill muffin papers and bake for 18 to 23 minutes, until golden brown. A toothpick in the center should come out clean.
6. Remove from the oven, and allow biscuits to cool for 5 to 10 minutes to encourage papers to come away from the biscuits. Serve warm or cold with buttery spread.

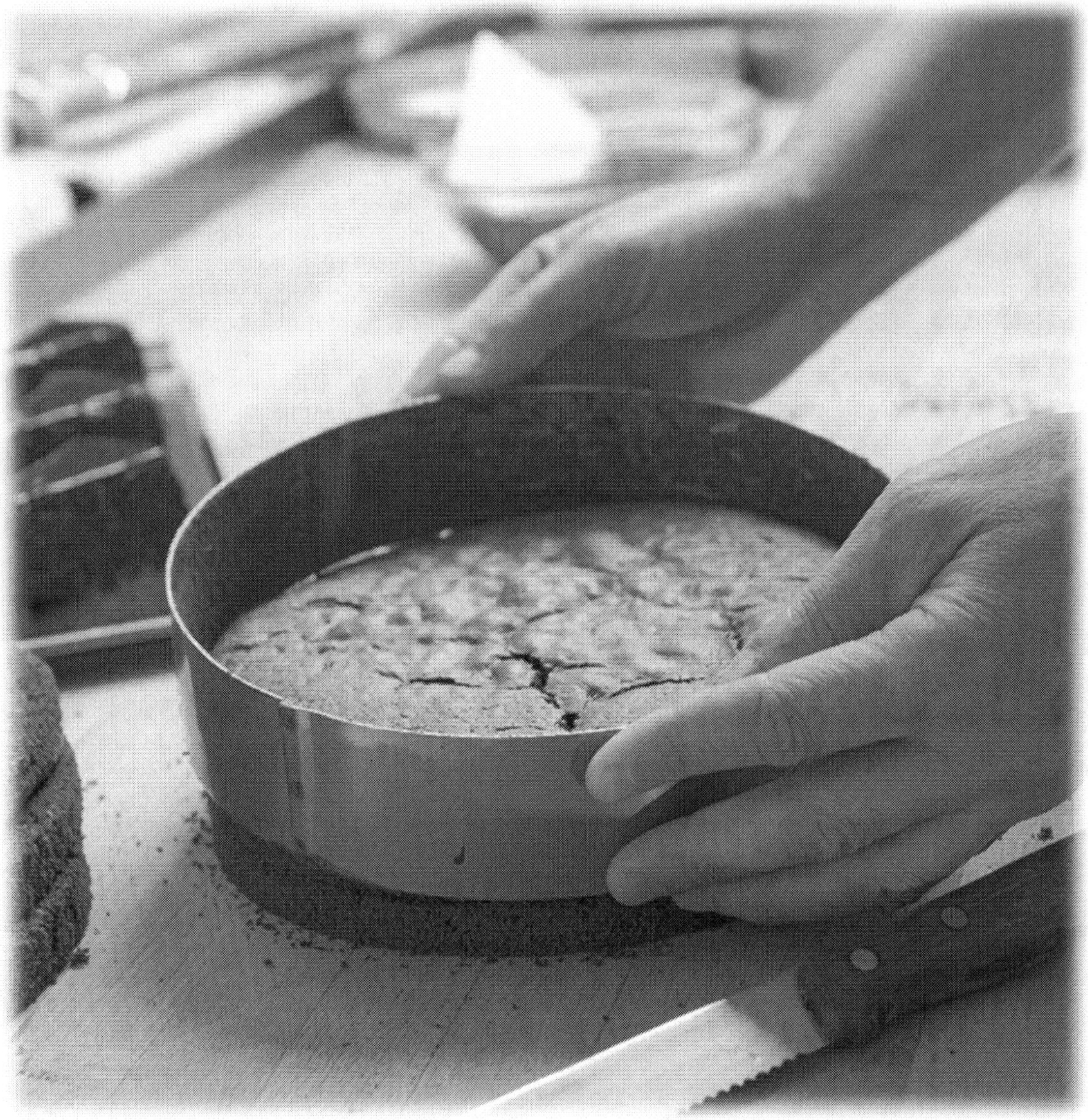

Cakes

Growing up in a Minnesota farm community, there was always cake in the house. Every farmer's wife had a number of great cake recipes, and the best recipes were freely traded. We could literally drop in at any farmhouse at 3:00 p.m. and be warmly greeted with fresh coffee and cake.

I thought designing numerous cake recipes would be, well, "a piece of cake," but I was so wrong because sugar not only makes baked goods sweet, it also creates volume and a light cake. That's why sugar is generally the second ingredient after flour in cake recipes. With the elimination of sugar and the substitution of vegetable glycerine and liquid stevia, no recipe responded in the way we expected, and the greatest challenge was to obtain and keep the lightness in those cake recipes that were supposed to be light.

The five recipes in this section are diverse in taste, texture, and appeal, so you're sure to find something that delights your palate. Our favorite is the Lemon Jellyroll, which never manages to make it past hour three out of the oven. Enjoy the sweetness between these pages!

Apple Streusel Coffee Cake

There is nothing like the sweet, warm cinnamon smell of coffee cake baking. This recipe came from a blend of ideas prompted by Bette Hagman's recipe for Swedish Coffee Cake in The Gluten-free Gourmet Cooks Comfort Foods, published by Henry Holt and Company, and the recipe for Streusel-filled Coffee Cake from Betty Crocker's New Picture Cookbook, published by McGraw Hill Book Company, circa 1961. Vegetable glycerine and liquid stevia are substituted for sugar, and coconut sugar is used in place of brown sugar. The addition of sliced apple rounds out the flavors, and makes this an exceptionally moist and delicious dessert. June

Serves: 6
Prep Time: 25 minutes
Bake Time: 65 minutes

Ingredients:

6 egg whites (retain 3 yolks)
3/4 teaspoon cream of tartar

---

1 1/2 cups Bette Hagman's Modified GF Flour Mix (see recipe in Mixes)
1 teaspoon baking soda
1 teaspoon xanthan gum
1/2 teaspoon salt

---

3 egg yolks
3 tablespoons vegetable glycerine
3 tablespoons oil
1 teaspoon SweetLeaf English Toffee liquid stevia

2/3 cup club soda

---

1 Gala or Braeburn apple peeled, cored and cut into thin slices

Streusel Mix:

3 tablespoons melted buttery spread

1/2 cup coconut sugar
2 teaspoons ground cinnamon

---

1 tablespoon coconut sugar

Kitchen Tools:

Stand or hand mixer

Medium and large mixer bowls

2 small bowls

Medium bowl

Measuring cups and spoons

8" x 8" baking pan

Large rubber spatula

Instructions:

1. Preheat oven to 350 degrees F (177 degrees C). Grease an 8" x 8" baking pan.
2. Separate eggs. Put egg whites and cream of tartar in a medium mixing bowl. Using a mixer, beat whites on low for 1 to 2 minutes to create small bubbles as a base. Increase mixer speed to high and beat until stiff peaks form.
3. In a larger mixing bowl, combine the flour mix, baking soda, xanthan gum, and salt. Stir well.
4. In a separate small bowl, beat the egg yolks, vegetable glycerine, oil, and liquid stevia. Add club soda and mix briefly. Pour into the flour mixture and beat until smooth. Mixture will thicken quickly, so, if necessary, be prepared to place the flat side of a rubber spatula just above the beaters to prevent batter from climbing into the beater mechanism.
5. Gently fold egg whites into batter by hand. A large spatula works most efficiently. Expect to see swirls of egg whites when completely folded in, so resist the urge to make the batter totally smooth, since stirring as opposed to folding will take the air out of egg whites.
6. Melt the buttery spread and set aside. In a small bowl, stir together coconut sugar and cinnamon.
7. Layer the various elements in this manner:
   - Arrange the apple slices in bottom of pan, single layer, fitting them together as you would a puzzle.
   - Drizzle with melted buttery spread over apples.
   - Sprinkle the streusel mix as evenly as possible over the apples.
   - Gently spread the batter over the streusel mix.
   - Sprinkle top with 1 tablespoon of coconut sugar.
8. Bake for 65 minutes. The toothpick test will not work with this recipe, so do not under bake. Serve warm or cold, with gooey, sweet apples on top.

Note: To double the recipe, use two 8" x 8" baking pans or the center will not bake properly.

Note: As with most gluten free baked goods without preservatives, this cake tends to become more solid and dry the next day. For best results and to improve texture, microwave for a few seconds to soften.

Variations:

Pear Streusel Coffee Cake: Substitute 1 peeled, sliced pear for the apple. Bake as directed.

Coconut Streusel Coffee Cake: Eliminate the apple and add 1/2 cup unsweetened shredded coconut to streusel mix. Reduce baking time to 60 minutes.

Marble Cake

Growing up in Midwestern farm country, Kris learned to make cakes at a young age when turning out a good cake was simple. However, gluten free, sugar-free cakes can be heavy due to the elimination of sugar. It took only two tries to get these sweet results. The vanilla portion uses vanilla stevia, and the chocolate portion is enhanced by chocolate raspberry stevia. This cake is moist, spongy, and needs no frosting. However, if you have gluten free, sugar free ice cream, you will have the perfect dessert. June

Serves: 6
Prep Time: 40 minutes
Bake Time: 35 to 45 minutes

Ingredients:
4 egg whites (retain the yolks)
1 teaspoon cream of tartar

Vanilla Part:
3/4 cup Bette Hagman's Featherlight Flour Mix (see recipe in Mixes)
2 tablespoons coconut flour
1 teaspoon baking soda
1/2 teaspoon xanthan gum
1/4 teaspoon salt

---

2 egg yolks
2 tablespoons vegetable glycerine
2 tablespoons oil
1 tablespoon Frontier Non-Alcoholic Vanilla
1 teaspoon SweetLeaf Vanilla Creme liquid Stevia

1/2 cup rice milk

Chocolate Part:
3/4 cup Bette Hagman's Featherlight Flour Mix (see recipe in Mixes)
2 tablespoons coconut flour
2 tablespoons cocoa
1 teaspoon baking soda
1/2 teaspoon xanthan gum
1/2 teaspoon cinnamon
1/4 plus 1/8 teaspoon salt

---

2 egg yolks
2 tablespoons vegetable glycerine
2 tablespoons oil
1 tablespoon Frontier Non-Alcoholic Vanilla
1 teaspoon SweetLeaf Chocolate Raspberry liquid Stevia

1/2 cup rice milk

Kitchen Tools:

Handheld mixer
2 medium mixer bowls
2 small bowls
Glass medium mixer bowl for egg whites
Measuring cups and spoons
8" x 8" baking pan

Instructions:

1. Preheat oven to 350 degrees F (177 degrees C). Grease an 8" x 8" baking pan.
2. Separate eggs. Put egg whites and cream of tartar in the glass bowl. Using a mixer, beat on low for 1 to 2 minutes to create small bubbles as a base. Increase mixer speed to high and beat until stiff peaks form. Set aside.
3. In two separate mixing bowls, combine the flour mix and dry ingredients for the vanilla part and chocolate part, keeping each separate. Stir to combine, breaking apart any lumps in soda, coconut flour, or flour mix.
4. In the small bowls, add the egg yolks, vegetable glycerine, oil, vanilla, and liquid stevias, keeping the vanilla and chocolate ingredients separate. Using the mixer, beat the contents of each bowl. Add the rice milk to each and beat briefly.
5. Working with the vanilla portion first, add the liquids to the flour mixture. Beat until smooth, at least 1 minute, scraping down the sides of the bowl.
6. Working with the chocolate portion next, mix the same way.
7. Place half the beaten egg whites onto the vanilla batter and the remainder onto the chocolate batter. Gently fold egg whites into each batter by hand. Expect to see swirls of egg whites when completely folded in, so resist the urge to make the batter totally smooth.
8. Pour one batter into the baking pan and gently spread around. Pour the other batter on top and, using a table knife, gently make swirls or zigzag movements through the batter to create the marbleized effect.
9. Bake for 35 to 45 minutes or until done. The toothpick test doesn't work with this recipe and individual ovens are different, so write down what timing works for you.

Whacky Cake

Home Economics Class in Underwood, Minnesota 50 years ago changed the way I looked at baking, and it was all because of Whacky Cake. I was amazed that a recipe with no milk or eggs could produce such a rich tasting, moist cake that needed no frosting. The beauty of the cake was that it could all be stirred up in the pan in which it was baked. That was my introduction to baking, and the fabulous results instantly had me hooked.

No one seems to know the origins of Whacky Cake, but it's believed to have come from the depression era when eggs and milk were scarce. Regardless of its source, it has always been a favorite for kids to make.

To get the same rich, moist, spongy chocolate results, we had to change every ingredient. We also added a bit of cinnamon to enhance the chocolate flavor and opted to use a mixer to combine all ingredients. June

Serves: 9
Prep Time: 25 minutes
Bake Time: 40 minutes

Ingredients:

1 1/4 cups Bette Hagman's Featherlight Flour Mix (see recipe in Mixes)
1/2 cup coconut flour
3 tablespoons cocoa powder
2 teaspoons baking soda
1 teaspoon xanthan gum
1 teaspoon ground cinnamon
3/4 teaspoon salt

1/2 cup grapeseed oil
1/4 cup fresh lemon juice (approximately 1 large lemon)
2 tablespoons Frontier Non-Alcoholic Vanilla

---

1 cup club soda
3 tablespoons vegetable glycerine
1 1/2 teaspoons SweetLeaf liquid stevia

Kitchen Tools:

Measuring cups and spoons

8" x 8" baking pan

Mixing bowl

Small bowl

Handheld mixer

Instructions:

1. Preheat oven to 350 degrees F (177 degrees C). Grease baking pan and set aside.
2. Measure the flours, cocoa powder, baking soda, xanthan gum, cinnamon, and salt into a mixing bowl. Stir until well combined.
3. Make three holes in the flour mixture. Pour the oil into one hole, lemon juice into the second hole, and vanilla into the third hole.
4. In a separate small bowl, mix the club soda, vegetable glycerine, and liquid stevia together. Pour over the top of batter. Mix well with a mixer.
5. Spread batter in the baking pan and bake for 40 minutes or until the center springs back when lightly touched or a toothpick comes out clean.
6. Serve warm or cold, plain or frosted with Chocolate Coconut Cream Frosting (see recipe in Sauces). This cake packs well in lunch boxes and stays moist.

Yellow Layer Cake

It was my grandson's 11th birthday, and he had been gluten free for a year and a half. He had become accustomed to celebrations not done in the unusual ways—holidays without traditional foods and birthdays without delicious birthday cakes when we were all working full-time. Careful planning was always required, as there was never a time when we had the option to pick up a sugar free, gluten free, dairy free birthday cake on the way home. For this birthday, I had the time to bake a cake, and this one became a new favorite for all of us.

The stiffened egg whites folded into the batter and the coconut flour give this cake its lightness. The vegetable glycerine and English Toffee liquid stevia make this cake sweet with a slightly nutty taste. June

Serves: 6 (because you'll want seconds)
Prep Time: 45 minutes
Bake Time: 60 minutes
Cooling Time: 45 minutes

Ingredients:
5 egg whites (retain yolks)
1 teaspoon cream of tartar

---

5 egg yolks
1/4 cup vegetable glycerine
1/4 cup oil
2 tablespoons Frontier Non-Alcoholic Vanilla
2 teaspoons SweetLeaf English Toffee liquid stevia

---

1 1/2 cups Bette Hagman's Featherlight Flour Mix (see recipe in Mixes)
1/2 cup coconut flour
1 1/2 teaspoons baking soda
1/2 teaspoon salt

---

1 1/2 cups rice milk
1 tablespoon cream of tartar

Kitchen Tools:

Handheld or stand mixer
Medium and large mixing bowl
Smaller bowl
Measuring cups and spoons
2-cup measuring cup or small bowl
Two 9" nonstick layer cake pans
Parchment paper

Instructions:

1. Preheat oven to 325 degrees F (163 degrees C). Cut 2 pieces of parchment paper the size of the bottom of your pans. Grease only the sides of the pans.
2. In a medium bowl and using a mixer, beat the egg whites and teaspoon of cream of tartar on low for 1 to 2 minutes. This will produce small bubbles as a base. Increase speed to high and beat until stiff peaks form. Set aside.
3. If you have a stand mixer, use it for the next step. There is no need to wash the beaters. Use a large mixing bowl and beat the egg yolks, vegetable glycerine, oil, vanilla, and liquid stevia for 1 minute.
4. In a small bowl, combine the featherlight flour, coconut flour, baking soda, and salt. Stir to mix well, making sure any chunks in the coconut flour are broken up. Add to the egg yolk mixture and mix well.
5. Measure the rice milk and tablespoon of cream of tartar into a 2-cup measuring cup or small bowl, and stir to dissolve. Add to the egg yolk mixture and beat for 1 minute.
6. Gently fold the egg whites into the batter by hand. A large spatula works best here. Expect to see 1/2" clumps of egg whites when entirely folded in, so resist the urge to make the batter smooth.
7. Evenly divide the batter between the two pans with the parchment paper in the bottom and smooth batter to the edges. Bake for 15 minutes, turn cake pans 180 degrees, and bake another 20 to 25 minutes or until center springs back when lightly touched.
8. Remove from oven and, using a plastic knife, loosen the edges of the cakes, gently flip over on a wire rack to cool, and remove the parchment paper. When entirely cooled, frost layers with Chocolate Coconut Cream Frosting, Sweet Berry Sauce (see recipes in Sauces), or sugar-free jam.

Tip: Store any leftover cake in the refrigerator, uncovered, to help maintain the cake's integrity.

Lemon Filled Jellyroll

I was first introduced to a homemade jellyroll in 1968. Until that time, it never occurred to me that these cakes didn't have to come out of a gooey cellophane wrapper, and my first taste of the real thing absolutely wowed me. When we went gluten free and sugar free, I became determined to recreate the jellyroll I loved, and this recipe does it.

The base was inspired by a recipe from the glutenfreeclub.com and ingredients were adjusted to suit our taste and allergies. The lemon filling was adapted from Betty Crocker's New Picture Cookbook, published by McGraw Hill Book Company, circa 1961. You can use anything you like between layers, as this jellyroll is very versatile, but, regardless of your choice, don't plan on this dessert making it to the second day. It's amazingly light tasting and totally addictive! My grandson declared the jellyroll was "defective" and graciously offered to eat it all. June

Serves: 4 (because you'll want seconds)
Prep Time: 50 minutes
Bake Time: 15 to 20 minutes
Cooling Time: 30 minutes

Jellyroll Ingredients:

3 egg whites (retain the yolks)
Dash of salt

---

3 egg yolks
1/4 cup vegetable glycerine
2 tablespoons finely grated lemon zest
2 teaspoons fresh lemon juice
1/2 teaspoon SweetLeaf liquid stevia

1/4 cup plus 1 tablespoon potato starch

Filling Ingredients:

1 1/2 cups water

1/4 cup cornstarch

3 tablespoons vegetable glycerine

1 1/8 teaspoons SweetLeaf liquid stevia

1/2 teaspoon SweetLeaf Lemon Drop liquid stevia

---

2 egg yolks, slightly beaten

---

2 tablespoons fresh grated lemon zest

3 tablespoons fresh lemon juice

1 tablespoon Frontier Non-Alcoholic Vanilla

Kitchen Tools:

Handheld or stand mixer

Measuring cups and spoons

Box grater for lemon zest

Citrus juicer

11" x 17" baking sheet

Parchment paper

Clean cotton dish towel (not terry cloth)

1 1/2-quart saucepan

Whisk

Instructions for Jellyroll:

1. Preheat oven to 325 degrees F (163 degrees C). Cut a piece of parchment paper the size of your pan and set aside. No need to grease the parchment paper.
2. Wash the lemon and, using the fine side of the grater, create enough lemon zest for the jellyroll and the filling. Juice the lemon and set aside.
3. Put egg whites and salt in a medium mixer bowl and with clean, dry beaters, beat on low for 1 minute. Increase speed to high and beat until stiff peaks form.
4. In a separate mixer bowl, beat the egg yolks, vegetable glycerine, 2 tablespoons lemon zest, 2 teaspoons lemon juice, and liquid stevia. Add potato starch and mix well.
5. Gently fold egg whites into egg yolk mixture with a rubber spatula. Expect to see 1/2" chunks of egg whites, so resist the urge to make the batter smooth.

6. Spread batter evenly in the pan over the parchment paper, making sure batter is of even thickness at each end. Bake for 15 to 20 minutes, until lightly tanned as opposed to browned, and the center springs back when gently touched.
7. Remove from oven and gently flip jellyroll onto clean dish towel. Carefully remove the parchment paper, and roll the towel and the jellyroll together the long way. Let cool for a half hour or so. Meanwhile, make the filling.

Instructions for Filling:

8. Stir the water, cornstarch, vegetable glycerine, and liquid stevias together in a saucepan until the cornstarch dissolves. Cook over medium heat, stirring constantly, until mixture thickens. Gently boil 1 minute.
9. In a separate bowl, whisk egg yolks until broken down. While whisking vigorously, pour at least half the hot mixture into the egg yolks. Return all to the saucepan and reducing heat a bit, boil for 1 minute longer, stirring constantly.
10. Remove from heat and stir in the lemon zest, lemon juice, and vanilla. Cool, stirring occasionally as it thickens, until the consistency is thick enough to spread.
11. To construct the jellyroll, gently unroll it from the towel. Spread filling evenly to within 1/2" of the edges to prevent filling from gooshing out. Reroll and slice with a serrated knife. Store loosely wrapped in plastic wrap.

Variations:

Mixed Berry Filling: Make a double batch of Sweet Berry Sauce (see recipe in Sauces). Follow remaining directions.

Chocolate Coconut Cream Filling: Use recipe for Chocolate Coconut Cream Frosting (see recipe in Sauces). Fill jellyroll just before serving. Refrigerate leftovers immediately.

Desserts

All our desserts were carefully developed with a balance of sugar-free sweetness. We began by experimenting with old comfort food recipes and designed brand new dishes. We tweaked ingredients, tried out new combinations of flavorings, threw away several failures, revamped, remade, and reinvented. Each success was celebrated.

A really good dessert can top off a meal, and in this section you will find puddings, pies, desserts that are baked, as well as some that need no baking. Be sure to try the Decadent Chocolate Mousse!

Bread Pudding

This is a great way to use up bread that has gone stale, or possibly a bread recipe that didn't turn out the way you expected. Any gluten-free bread will be given new life that even children will enjoy. Bread pudding is great as a dessert or an easy breakfast.

Some recipes are more difficult than others to get right, and this recipe consistently evaded perfection. We joyfully ate all the failures and celebrated when the elements of flavor, richness, and texture finally came together. We prefer it served cold with a dollop of chilled coconut cream on top. June

Serves: 6
Prep Time: 30 minutes
Bake Time: 55 to 65 minutes

Ingredients:

2 cups rice milk
1 cup coconut milk
3 tablespoons vegetable glycerine
1 teaspoon SweetLeaf English Toffee liquid stevia
1/4 teaspoon salt

---

3 eggs
2 tablespoons Bette Hagman's Featherlight Flour Mix (see recipe in Mixes)
2 tablespoons Frontier Non-Alcoholic Vanilla
1 tablespoon Egg Replacer

---

2 cups gluten-free bread, cut into 3/8" cubes

Kitchen Tools:

2 1/2-quart saucepan

Handheld mixer or whisk

Medium mixer bowl

8" x 8" baking dish

Shallow pan large enough for baking dish to fit into with enough space for hot water

Instructions:

1. Preheat oven to 350 degrees F (177 degrees C). Oil an 8" x 8" baking dish and set aside.
2. Heat rice milk, coconut milk, vegetable glycerine, liquid stevia, and salt in the saucepan just until it bubbles around the edges.
3. In a medium mixing bowl, beat together eggs, flour, vanilla, and egg replacer. Slowly pour milk mixture into eggs and beat until well combined.
4. Stir bread bits into the milk and egg mixture and pour into baking dish. Place baking dish into larger pan and pour enough hot water into larger pan so an inch of inner pan is sitting in the water.
5. Bake for 55 to 65 minutes. Remove from oven and keep in hot water for 20 minutes. Remove pudding pan from the outer pan and cool on a rack. Custard may not appear to be set, using the standard "knife inserted in the center coming out clean" test, but dessert will further set as it cools.
6. Refrigerate and serve cold with chilled coconut cream, if desired.

Tip: To double recipe, put in two separate 8" x 8" baking dishes.

Tip: To easily add boiling water to outer pan, pour hot water through a funnel.

Chocolate Pudding

When I Googled what percentage of people don't like chocolate, I came up with no credible studies but an estimate of "a very small percentage." I would agree with that, and for most of us, a good chocolate dish offers a great deal of satisfaction.

This pudding fills that "chocolate hole" most of us were born with. This sweet, thick, and creamy easy-to-make pudding is sure to please, and totally kid approved. June

Makes: 3 cups

Prep Time: 5 minutes

Cook Time: 15 minutes

Cooling Time: At least 1 hour

Ingredients:

2 eggs beaten

1 cup cold rice milk

1/2 cup cornstarch

1/2 cup cocoa powder

1/4 cup vegetable glycerine

1 teaspoon SweetLeaf Chocolate liquid stevia

1/2 teaspoon salt

1/2 teaspoon xanthan gum

1/4 teaspoon SweetLeaf Chocolate Raspberry liquid stevia

---

1 cup rice milk

1 cup coconut milk

---

1 tablespoon Frontier Non-Alcoholic Vanilla

Kitchen Tools:

Wire whisk

1 1/2-quart saucepan or larger

Medium sized bowl

Measuring cups and spoons

Blender

Instructions:

1. Place eggs, 1 cup of rice milk, cornstarch, cocoa powder, vegetable glycerine, liquid stevias, salt, and xanthan gum in a blender, and blend on high for at least 1 minute, dissolving ingredients into milk. Pour into saucepan and stir in the remaining rice milk and coconut milk.
2. Heat over medium heat, stirring constantly. As mixture gets thick, stir with enthusiasm to prevent lumps. Boil 1 minute.
3. Remove from heat and stir in the vanilla.
4. Cool at least one hour before serving, but pudding tastes best when served cold with a dollop of chilled coconut cream on top. Cool uncovered in refrigerator for 24 hours and then cover.

Variations:

Dark Chocolate Pudding: Replace 1 tablespoon of the cocoa powder with 1 tablespoon dark chocolate cocoa powder. Cook as directed.

Rice Milk Chocolate Pudding: Substitute 1 cup of rice milk for the coconut milk and increase xanthan gum to 3/4 teaspoon.

Mexican Chocolate Pudding: Add 1/2 teaspoon cinnamon in step 1 of the process. Garnish with shaved chocolate, whipped coconut cream, fresh raspberries or all of the above.

Vanilla Pudding

This pudding is rich, thick, and creamy even when served warm. My young son said it was better than the boxed pudding he had made!

This recipe was inspired by Betty Crocker's New Picture Cookbook, published by McGraw Hill Book Company, circa 1961, from which I first learned to cook. This awesome book taught young women the fine art of being a homemaker, including how to set a table for tea, host a party, and make radish roses and carrot curls. It also addressed quality of life issues such as combing you hair and putting on make-up and perfume for you and your family's morale! In fact, we've used this book so much over the years before our food allergies kicked in, that the binding is missing and the pages are yellowed with age. It is always nice to bring back an old friend!

So sit back, relax, and enjoy this sweet pudding with a cup of coffee or your favorite tea and a good book. It's great warm or chilled. Kris

Makes: 2 cups
Prep time: 5 minutes
Cook Time: 10 to 15 minutes
Cooling Time: 2 hours or more

Ingredients:

2 cups rice milk
1/4 cup plus 1 tablespoon cornstarch
1 tablespoon vegetable glycerine
1/2 teaspoon SweetLeaf Apricot Nectar liquid stevia
1/4 teaspoon SweetLeaf Vanilla Creme liquid stevia
1/4 teaspoon salt

---

2 eggs, well beaten

---

2 tablespoons Frontier Non-Alcoholic Vanilla

Kitchen Tools:

2-quart saucepan

Measuring cups and spoons

Medium sized bowl

Handheld mixer or whisk

Instructions:

1. Stir the rice milk, cornstarch, vegetable glycerine, stevias, and salt together in a saucepan until cornstarch is dissolved.
2. Cook over medium heat, stirring constantly, until mixture thickens. Boil 1 minute and remove from heat. Mixture will be thick.
3. Break eggs into a medium bowl and, using a whisk or handheld mixer, mix well.
4. While still mixing, gradually pour at least half the hot rice milk mixture into the beaten eggs. Pour the egg mixture back into the saucepan. Continuing to stir and heat just until it comes to a boil.
5. Remove from heat, stir in vanilla and chill in the refrigerator uncovered, if serving cold.
6. Once pudding has cooled, garnish with chilled coconut cream, whipped coconut cream, fresh fruit, coconut shavings, gluten/soy/dairy free chocolate chips, or anything else that makes it even more special.

Variations:

Butterscotch: In step 1, substitute 1/2 teaspoon SweetLeaf English Toffee liquid stevia for the Apricot Nectar liquid stevia. Reduce vanilla to 1 tablespoon.

Lemon: In step 1, substitute 1/2 teaspoon SweetLeaf Lemon Drop liquid stevia for the Apricot Nectar liquid stevia. Stir in 1 tablespoon fresh lemon zest with the vanilla.

Cookies and Cream: Crumble your favorite gluten-free cookie into the cooked, chilled pudding.

Nutless Toffee Pudding

I was in a creative mood and, since I love a challenge, a container of roasted pumpkin seeds presented just the right ingredient for experimentation. This pudding begins with a finely-processed pumpkin seed paste that is wonderfully sweet. When combined with the liquids and cooked, the natural flavors are released and the pudding becomes a combination of smoothness and texture.

This is a rich, high-protein food, and a little bit goes a long way toward satisfaction. We found it to be a great breakfast that held us through until lunchtime. Kris

Makes: 2 1/2 cups
Prep Time: 25 minutes
Cook Time: 5 minutes
Cooling Time: At least 1 hour

Pumpkin Seed Paste Ingredients:

1/2 cup roasted shelled pumpkin seeds

---

2 tablespoons melted coconut oil
1 tablespoon vegetable glycerine
1 tablespoon Frontier Non-Alcoholic Vanilla
1/8 teaspoon salt
6 drops SweetLeaf English Toffee liquid stevia

Pudding Ingredients:

1 1/4 cups rice milk
1 cup coconut milk

---

2 egg yolks
2 tablespoons cornstarch
1 teaspoon vegetable glycerine
1/4 teaspoon SweetLeaf English Toffee liquid stevia
1/8 teaspoon salt

---

3 tablespoons Frontier Non-Alcoholic Vanilla

Kitchen Tools:

Small food processor

Measuring cups and spoons

2-quart saucepan

Whisk

Handheld mixer

Small bowl

Instructions:

1. Place pumpkin seeds in the food processor and pulse until seeds are in small pieces. Add coconut oil, vegetable glycerine, vanilla, salt and liquid stevia. Process on high for 2 minutes.
2. Place pumpkin seed paste in saucepan and gradually stir in the rice milk and coconut milk. Whisk over medium heat and gently boil for 30 seconds. If mixture curdles, don't be concerned. It will reintegrate in the next step.
3. Using a handheld mixer, beat together in a small bowl the egg yolks, cornstarch, vegetable glycerine, stevia, and salt. While still beating, pour about half the hot mixture into the egg yolks and, if the heated combination has curdled, pour the remainder into the bowl, mixing well. Return mixture to the saucepan.
4. Heat pudding over medium heat, stirring constantly, until thick and bubbly. Boil for 1 minute.
5. Remove from heat and stir in vanilla. Cool completely and refrigerate. Serve cold.

Baked Rice Custard

Baked rice pudding is a great way to satisfy a sweet tooth, guilt free. The end product is best served cold with a dollop of chilled coconut cream on top. Coconut cream can be found in cans in the oriental section of most grocery stores.

This recipe was adapted from the Custard Rice Pudding recipe in Betty Crocker's New Picture Cookbook, published by McGraw Hill Book Company, circa 1961. Even 50 years later, baked custards of any kind are still considered a comfort food. This dish can be a wonderful ending to a meal or a quick, satisfying breakfast. June

Serves: 4 (you'll want large servings)
Prep Time: 25 minutes
Bake Time: 1 hour 25 minutes
Cooling Time: 1 hour or more

Ingredients:

1 1/2 cups coconut milk
1 1/2 cups rice milk

---

5 eggs, beaten
1/4 cup vegetable glycerine
1 1/2 tablespoons Frontier Non-Alcoholic Vanilla
3/4 teaspoon SweetLeaf English Toffee liquid stevia
3/4 teaspoon salt
1/2 teaspoon nutmeg

---

1 cup cooked white rice (preferably basmati or jasmine)

Kitchen Tools:

Medium bowl

Handheld mixer or whisk

2-quart saucepan

Measuring cups and spoons

8" x 8" glass baking dish

Shallow pan large enough for baking dish with enough space for hot water

Instructions:

1. Preheat oven to 350 degrees F (177 degrees C). Oil baking dish and set aside.
2. Heat coconut milk and rice milk over medium to medium high heat in a saucepan, just to the boiling point. Stir occasionally to ensure that it doesn't burn.
3. In a medium sized bowl, using handheld mixer or whisk, beat together eggs, vegetable glycerine, vanilla, liquid stevia, salt, and nutmeg. When milk mixture is hot, slowly pour milk into egg mixture, beating constantly.
4. Stir cooked rice into mixture, and pour into glass baking dish.
5. Place baking dish into the larger pan and pour enough hot water into the outer pan so at least an inch of the glass baking dish is sitting in the water. An easy way to accomplish this is to pour the hot water through a funnel.
6. Bake on center rack of your oven for 1 hour 25 minutes or until a table knife inserted into the center comes out "uncoated." Remove from oven and cool on a rack. This custard is best served cold.

Decadent Chocolate Mousse

Even though I have severe food allergies, there are a couple of restaurants in our local area in which we can dine, as long as we let the waitperson know which foods I need to avoid. At best, I usually have one item on any menu that I can safely consume, and I count myself as blessed if I have two choices. Some restaurants are more allergy-conscious than others, and Great Sage in Clarksville, Maryland does a wonderful job of meeting the needs of people with allergies. It's a vegan restaurant and all menu items are identified by each common allergen in that dish. Most dishes are offered with soy and gluten-free alternatives.

They offer an outstanding chocolate mousse, with agave nectar as the sweetener. Since agave is too sweet for my body, we decided to see if we could recreate this dish from taste bud memory. We fiddled with the base, the proportions, and ingredients until we hit upon this combination.

This dessert is so velvety smooth and rich, no one will ever suspect it is healthy and made of ripe avocados! It is very dense, so you will find that just a little bit is remarkably satisfying. Best served cold, we think you'll love the taste and texture as much as we do. Kris

Serves: 4 adults and a small child
Prep Time: 30 minutes
Cook Time: 5 minutes

Ingredients:

2 tablespoons coconut milk
1 tablespoon coconut oil
2 1/2 teaspoons vegetable glycerine
1 1/4 teaspoons SweetLeaf Vanilla Creme liquid stevia

1/4 cup plus 2 tablespoons cocoa powder

---

1 cup ripe avocado, mashed

---

3 tablespoons Frontier Non-Alcoholic Vanilla
1/8 teaspoon sea salt

Kitchen Tools:

Small saucepan

Small food processor

Measuring cup and spoons

Instructions:

1. In a small saucepan, gently melt together the coconut oil, coconut milk, stevia, and vegetable glycerine. Stir in the cocoa powder, and continue to cook gently, stirring constantly, for about 30 seconds. Remove from heat and let cool slightly. It will be thick.
2. Remove the meat of the ripe avocado and measure out 1 cup. Process in food processor for 1 minute or until smooth.
3. Add chocolate mixture, vanilla, and salt to avocado and process for another minute on high, scraping down the sides of the processor until smooth. Refrigerate at least an hour to allow the flavors to marry and for the consistency to firm up.
4. Serve cold in small servings plain or with a dollop of chilled coconut cream. The mousse is wonderfully rich, so small servings will be very satisfying. If you can detect a slight taste of the avocado base, refrigerate overnight.

Variations:

Mexican Chocolate Mousse: In step 1, add 1 1/2 teaspoons ground cinnamon. Follow remaining directions.

Black Raspberry Mousse: In place of the vanilla creme liquid stevia, substitute 3/4 teaspoon SweetLeaf Chocolate Raspberry liquid stevia and 1/2 teaspoon SweetLeaf plain liquid stevia. Follow remaining directions.

Chocolate Orange Cinnamon Mousse: Add 1/2 teaspoon cinnamon, 3/4 teaspoon SweetLeaf Valentia Orange liquid stevia and 1/2 teaspoon SweetLeaf Vanilla Creme liquid stevia.

Lemon Bars

These Lemon Bars were the result of my craving for something lemon, sweet, and much simpler to make than lemon meringue pie. This was one of those ideas we toyed with, systemically trying new combinations or tweaking quantities and elements, and at the end of two years, we had reached the taste and texture we wanted.

This recipe calls for lucuma powder, which is finely milled whole Peruvian lucuma fruit that has been dried at low temperatures. Lucuma powder is a low glycemic natural sweetener that contains nutrients such as vitamin B3, iron, zinc, beta-carotene, calcium, and protein. The flavor is best described as a prunish-malty taste that blends with and accents the ingredients in this crust. The coconut nectar is a sweet, low glycemic syrup, which can be found in health food stores and some grocery stores. June

Serves: 12
Prep Time: 50 minutes
Bake Time: 50 minutes

Shortbread Crust Ingredients:

1 1/4 cups Bette Hagman's Modified GF Flour Mix (see recipe in Mixes)
1 tablespoon lucuma powder
1/2 teaspoon xanthan gum
1/2 teaspoon ground cinnamon
1/4 teaspoon salt

1/4 cup buttery spread
1 tablespoon Frontier Non-Alcoholic Vanilla
1 tablespoon vegetable glycerine
1 1/2 teaspoons coconut nectar
1/4 teaspoon SweetLeaf English Toffee liquid stevia

Filling Ingredients:

2 tablespoons lemon zest
1/4 cup plus 2 tablespoons fresh lemon juice (approximately 1 1/2 lemons)

---

2 cups water
1/3 cup plus 2 tablespoons cornstarch
1/4 cup vegetable glycerine
3 tablespoons tapioca syrup
1 teaspoon SweetLeaf liquid stevia
3/4 teaspoon SweetLeaf Lemon Drop liquid stevia

---

4 egg yolks

---

2 tablespoons Frontier Non-Alcoholic Vanilla

Kitchen Tools:

8" x 8" baking dish
Measuring cups and spoons
Box grater
Citrus juicer
Medium sized bowl
Whisk or handheld mixer
Small bowl
Small skillet

Crust Instructions:

1. Preheat oven to 350 degrees F (177 degrees C). Oil baking dish and set aside.
2. In a medium sized bowl, stir together the flour mix, lucuma powder, xanthan gum, cinnamon, and salt.
3. In a small bowl, mix together the buttery spread, vanilla, vegetable glycerine, coconut nectar, and stevia. Combine dry and wet ingredients and stir until mixed well.
4. Press the dough into the baking pan, forming an even base, and prick the dough with a fork every inch or so.
5. Bake crust for 15 minutes or until lightly browned. Set aside on a rack to cool while you make the filling.

Filling Instructions:

6. Preheat oven again to 350 degrees F (177 degrees C).
7. Wash lemon(s) and create lemon zest using a fairly fine side of a grater. Measure out 2 tablespoons and set aside. Juice the lemon(s) and measure juice, adding it to the lemon zest.
8. In a medium sized saucepan, mix the water, cornstarch, vegetable glycerine, tapioca syrup, and liquid stevias until cornstarch is dissolved. Stirring constantly over medium heat, boil 1 minute.
9. In a medium bowl, beat egg yolks until broken down. Slowly pour hot liquid into egg yolks while mixing constantly. Pour back into saucepan and continue to stir while boiling for 1 minute longer.
10. Remove from heat and stir in lemon juice, lemon zest, and vanilla. Spread evenly over crust and bake for 50 minutes. Remove from oven, cool on a rack, and refrigerate until thoroughly chilled. The flavor is best when served cold.

Note: There's a fine balance of flavors and sweeteners designed into this recipe. As a result, the filling, if tasted alone, has an aftertaste. When eaten with the crust base, the flavors will wow your taste buds.

Note: For a special treat, serve with your favorite vanilla non-dairy ice cream.

Crumb Pie Crust

The inspiration for this recipe was a failed batch of lemon shortbread cookies. Coming from a frugal, German heritage, the idea of seeing the cookies in the trash simply was not an option. It occurred to me that the cookies could be ground up and used as the base for a crumb crust. This pie crust is wonderfully versatile, and can be used with almost any sweet filling. If you don't have lemon cookies to grind up, gluten free graham crackers will do nicely. June

Makes: 1 crust
Prep Time: 10 minutes
Bake Time: 7 minutes

Ingredients:

1 1/2 cups finely ground gluten free lemon cookie crumbs or "graham" crackers
1/2 teaspoon ground cinnamon
1/4 teaspoon salt

---

3 tablespoons buttery spread
1 tablespoon vegetable glycerine
1/4 teaspoon SweetLeaf Cinnamon liquid stevia

Kitchen Tools:

9" pie pan
Measuring spoons and cups
Stirring spoon
Mixing bowl
Small bowl

Instructions:

1. Preheat oven to 375 degrees F (191 degrees C).
2. Grind cookies or "graham" crackers to make 1 1/2 cups and put in a bowl. Stir in the cinnamon and salt.
3. In a small bowl, combine buttery spread, vegetable glycerine, and liquid stevia. Add to crumb mixture and thoroughly blend with a spoon. Mixture should be crumbly but hold together when pressed.
4. Pour into pie pan and press into the bottom and sides to form a crust of uniform density. Bake for 7 minutes. When cooled, fill with your choice of filling that does not have to be baked.

Notta Kolache

When Kris was three years old, we moved to Strasburg, North Dakota, the hometown of Lawrence Welk. It was a German-Russian community, rich with mixed culture, and a blend of the two languages could be heard more often than English. One of the pastries I loved was called Kuchen, a sweet, raised dough baked with a rich custard on top. Even 40 years later, I still remember the taste.

I was delighted when a Czech bakery opened down the road and their specialty was Kolache. My first taste of Kolache brought back a flood of memories of Kuchen and I determined to reconstruct the same taste, gluten free and without yeast. After several attempts, I had to concede that some things just may not be able to be duplicated in a way we can all enjoy. Kris suggested going a different direction entirely, with a chocolate brownie base but keeping the custard topping, and it turned out to be a perfect combination when drizzled with Caramel Syrup. We decided to call it Notta Kolache. June

Serves: 8

Prep Time: 45 minutes

Bake Time: 35 minutes

Chocolate Base Ingredients:

2 eggs
1/2 cup any gluten free flour blend
1/2 cup plus 2 tablespoons cocoa powder
1/2 cup grapeseed oil
3 tablespoons coconut flour
3 tablespoons vegetable glycerine
2 tablespoons rice milk
1 tablespoon Frontier Non-Alcoholic Vanilla
3/4 teaspoon salt
3/4 teaspoon SweetLeaf Chocolate liquid stevia
3/4 teaspoon SweetLeaf Chocolate Raspberry liquid stevia
1/2 teaspoon ground cinnamon

Custard Ingredients:

1 1/2 cups coconut milk
3/4 cup rice milk
3 tablespoons cornstarch
3 tablespoons vegetable glycerine
3/4 teaspoon SweetLeaf English Toffee liquid stevia
1/8 teaspoon salt

---

3 eggs

---

1 tablespoon Frontier Non-Alcoholic Vanilla

Caramel Syrup:

1/4 cup tapioca syrup

3/4 teaspoon SweetLeaf English Toffee liquid stevia

Kitchen Tools:

2 1/2-quart saucepan

8" x 8" baking dish

Whisk or handheld mixer

Measuring cups and spoons

Medium bowl

Small bowl

Instructions for Chocolate Base:

1. Preheat oven to 325 degrees F (163 degrees C). Oil baking dish and set aside.
2. Put all ingredients for the chocolate base in a mixing bowl and blend until smooth, scraping down the sides of the bowl. Spread batter evenly in the baking dish and set aside while you make the custard topping.

Instructions for Custard Topping:

3. In a saucepan, stir together the coconut milk, rice milk, cornstarch, vegetable glycerine, liquid stevia, and salt until cornstarch is dissolved. Heat over medium heat and boil 1 minute, stirring constantly.
4. Break eggs into a medium bowl and with a whisk or handheld mixer. Beat well. Slowly pour hot custard into the eggs while still beating vigorously, and then pour mixture back into saucepan.
5. Return the pan to medium heat and bring just to a boil. Stir in vanilla and gently pour custard over the chocolate base, spreading evenly.
6. Bake for 35 minutes and allow to cool on a rack. Meanwhile, stir the tapioca syrup and liquid stevia together and set aside at room temperature.
7. When Notta Kolache is thoroughly cooled, cut with a knife dipped in cold water, and serve with caramel syrup drizzled over. Refrigerate leftovers, loosely covered.

Tip: Tapioca syrup should be refrigerated after opening. To soften, place jar in hot water for a few minutes. Do not microwave as it will turn the syrup into a fairly solid, sticky mass.

Chocolate Pie

Chocolate Pie is a comfort food and standard fare in diners and small, Midwestern town cafes of long ago. It's a simple pleasure of taste and texture that is smooth and cool on the tongue, with a crust that melts in the mouth.

And then there's the chocolate factor. I personally believe chocolate should be classified as an essential food group—right up there with proteins and vegetables. This is a rich chocolate, with just a hint of raspberry, effortlessly achieved by using chocolate raspberry liquid stevia. Teamed up with a standard pie crust or a crumb crust, this dessert is kid approved and sure to satisfy young and old. June

Serves: 6
Prep Time: 5 minutes
Cook Time: 15 minutes
Cooling Time: At least 1 hour

Ingredients:

Prepared pie crust

---

2 cups cold rice milk
1 cup cold coconut milk
1/2 cup plus 1 tablespoon cornstarch
1/3 cup plus 2 tablespoons cocoa powder
1/4 cup vegetable glycerine
3/4 teaspoon SweetLeaf Chocolate Raspberry liquid stevia
1/2 teaspoon salt
1/2 teaspoon xanthan gum

---

2 eggs beaten

---

2 tablespoons Frontier Non-Alcoholic Vanilla

Kitchen Tools:

Wire whisk

1 1/2-quart saucepan or larger

Medium sized bowl

Measuring cups and spoons

Blender

Pie pan

Instructions:

1. Prepare and bake a single pie crust (see recipe in this section) and set aside.
2. Pour rice milk, coconut milk, cornstarch, cocoa powder, vegetable glycerine, liquid stevia, salt, and xanthan gum in blender. Blend on high to dissolve ingredients into milk. Pour into saucepan and heat over medium heat, stirring constantly until smooth and very thick.
3. In a medium sized bowl, whisk eggs until well beaten. While still whisking vigorously, dollop about half the hot mixture into the eggs, and then pour back into the saucepan, stirring vigorously.
4. Continue to cook, stirring constantly for 1 minute. Remove from heat and stir in the vanilla.
5. Cool at least 1/2 hour before pouring into pie crust. Chill thoroughly before cutting. To store, cover loosely with plastic wrap and refrigerate.

Variations:

Dark Chocolate Filling: Replace 1 tablespoon of the cocoa powder with 1 tablespoon of dark chocolate cocoa powder. Cook as directed.

Lemon Meringue Pie

Do you love lemon meringue pie but haven't found a recipe that is sugar free, gluten free, and still tastes good? This is a traditional lemon meringue pie, using only fresh ingredients. As we have discovered, there are no short cuts to great lemon meringue pie. Don't try to cut your time by using bottled lemon juice or dried lemon zest—you'll only be disappointed. While this dessert takes a bit of time, the results are so worth it. June

Serves: 6
Prep Time: 55 minutes
Cook Time: 15 minutes
Bake Time: 4 to 6 minutes
Cooling Time: 1 hour or more

Lemon Filling Ingredients:

Prepared, single pie crust, baked (see recipe in this section)

---

1 tablespoon grated lemon zest
1/4 cup fresh squeezed lemon juice

---

1 1/2 cups cool water
1/3 cup cornstarch
1/4 cup tapioca syrup
3 tablespoons vegetable glycerine
1 teaspoon SweetLeaf Lemon Drop liquid stevia
1/4 teaspoon salt

---

3 beaten egg yolks (retain egg whites for meringue)

Meringue Ingredients:

3 egg whites
1/4 teaspoon cream of tartar

---

1 tablespoon Frontier Non-Alcoholic Vanilla
1 tablespoon vegetable glycerine
3/4 teaspoon liquid stevia

Kitchen Tools:

9" pie pan
Measuring spoons and cups
Citrus juicer
Box grater
Handheld mixer
1 1/2-quart saucepan
Mixing bowls
Fork or whisk

Lemon Filling Instructions:

1. Wash lemon and, using a fairly fine side of the grater, make lemon zest. Measure out 1 tablespoon and set aside. Juice the lemon and set aside.
2. In a saucepan, combine water, cornstarch, tapioca syrup, vegetable glycerine, liquid stevia, and salt. Stir until cornstarch dissolves and cook over medium heat until bubbly, stirring constantly. Boil 1 minute.
3. Separate the eggs, putting the yolks into a small bowl and the whites in a glass mixing bowl for the meringue. Set whites aside. With a whisk or handheld mixer, break down the egg yolks until well mixed.
4. While continuing to whisk the egg yolks, pour at least half the hot liquid into the egg yolks. Pour this mixture back into the saucepan and return to medium heat. Boil 1 minute, stirring constantly.
5. Remove from heat and stir in the lemon juice and lemon zest. Set aside but keep hot while you make the meringue.

Meringue Instructions:

6. If you have just used your beaters for the egg yolks, wash them with soap and hot water to remove all oil. Rinse and dry thoroughly. With a mixer, beat egg whites and cream of tartar on low for 1 minute. Turn mixer on high and continue to beat until soft peaks form. Add vanilla, vegetable glycerine, and liquid stevia. Continue to beat on high until stiff peaks form.
7. Preheat oven to 400 degrees F (204 degrees C). Pour hot filling into pie crust. Spread the meringue on the hot filling making sure the meringue reaches the edges of the crust to seal the filling. If there's a gap between meringue and crust, the meringue will shrink as it cools. Make swirls in the meringue to add artistic value. Bake for 6 minutes until lightly browned but check every minute after 4 minutes, as the vegetable glycerine will cause the meringue to get overly brown quickly.
8. Cool thoroughly before cutting. Store any leftover pieces in the refrigerator, uncovered.

Tip: To make lemon zest, wash the lemon using a bit of dish soap, rinse well, and pat dry. When grating the lemon, under no circumstance should you juice the lemon first and then try to grate the rind. If you do, have a Band-Aid ready—you'll need it. When measuring lemon zest, loosely pack in your measuring spoon.

Sweet Potato Pie

The differences between pumpkin pie and sweet potato pie are subtle, and, although Mom has no preference, I definitely prefer sweet potato pie. As I defined it for her, sweet potatoes are sweeter with a smoother texture while pumpkin has a courser flavor. Put another way, pumpkin is clearly a vegetable and sweet potato is a delectable dessert.

In place of the usual brown sugar, we have used a combination of liquid stevia, vegetable glycerine, and brown rice syrup. Even if you've never had sweet potato pie, give this recipe a try. Kris

Serves: 6
Prep Time: 30 minutes
Bake Time: 1 hour 30 minutes
Cooling Time: 1 hour or longer

Ingredients:

Prepared, single unbaked 9" pie crust (see recipe in this section)

---

1 egg
1 15-oz. can sweet potatoes or 1 1/2 cups of fresh, cooked and pureed
1/4 cup plus 2 tablespoons buttery spread
3 tablespoons brown rice syrup
2 tablespoons vegetable glycerine
3/4 teaspoon ground cinnamon
1/2 teaspoon ground nutmeg
1/4 teaspoon SweetLeaf English Toffee liquid stevia
1/8 teaspoon salt

1/3 cup coconut milk
2 tablespoons Frontier Non-Alcoholic Vanilla

Kitchen Tools:

9" pie pan

Stand or handheld mixer

Measuring cups and spoons

Aluminum foil

Instructions:

1. Preheat oven to 400 degrees F (204 degrees C).
2. In a mixing bowl, combine egg, sweet potato, buttery spread, brown rice syrup, vegetable glycerine, cinnamon, nutmeg, liquid stevia, and salt. Beat on high for 1 minute.
3. Add coconut milk and vanilla, and mix well.
4. Pour into pie crust and cover the exposed edge of crust with aluminum foil. Bake at 400 degrees F (204 degrees C) for 10 minutes. Reduce heat to 350 degrees F (177 degrees C) and bake for 1 hour. Remove foil and bake for another 20 minutes.
5. Remove from oven and cool before serving.

Very Berry Cobbler

Cobblers are an American deep-dish dessert or pie, usually with a biscuit crust and a fruit filling, such as peaches, apples, or berries. The term cobbler derives from "cobble up," meaning to throw together in a hurry.

The inspiration for this dessert came from a Blackberry Cobbler recipe in Gluten-free, Sugar-free Cooking by Susan O'Brien, copyright 2006, published by Da Capo Press. The original recipe was a huge success in our house, but as we developed multiple food allergies, we needed to rework the recipe yet still maintain the same, wonderful taste. The end result is a no-guilt, healthy, sweet cobbler that can be served just as easily for breakfast or a dinner dessert. This passed the kid test with requests for seconds! June

Serves: 8

Prep Time: 35 minutes

Bake Time: 30 minutes

Berry Base Ingredients:

5 cups fresh blackberries, raspberries and blueberries, washed and drained

1/4 cup vegetable glycerine

2 tablespoons brown rice flour

1 tablespoon Frontier Non-Alcoholic Vanilla

1/2 teaspoon SweetLeaf liquid stevia

12 drops Frontier Alcohol Free Orange flavoring

Cobbler Ingredients:

1/2 cup coconut milk, at least 17% fat per 1/2 cup

2 eggs

---

2 tablespoons buttery spread, melted

1 tablespoon vegetable glycerine

1 tablespoon Frontier Non-Alcoholic Vanilla

1/4 teaspoon SweetLeaf liquid stevia

6 drops Frontier Alcohol Free Orange flavoring

---

1 cup brown rice flour

2 teaspoons Baking Powder (see recipe in Mixes)

1/2 teaspoon salt

---

1 1/2 tablespoons coconut sugar

Kitchen Tools:

Small bowl

Medium sized mixing bowl

Measuring cups and spoons

8" x 11" baking dish

Whisk or handheld mixer

Instructions:

1. Preheat oven to 400 degrees F (204 degrees C). Oil baking dish and set aside.
2. Gently stir together the berries, vegetable glycerine, brown rice flour, vanilla, liquid stevia, and orange flavor. Spread evenly in the baking dish.
3. In a medium sized bowl, using a whisk or mixer, combine coconut milk and eggs. Add the buttery spread, vegetable glycerine, vanilla, liquid stevia, and orange flavoring.
4. In a small bowl, stir together the 1 cup brown rice flour, baking powder, and salt. Add to the coconut milk mixture and stir just until mixed. Do not over mix.
5. Drop by tablespoons on fruit mixture, as evenly as possible. Sprinkle with coconut sugar.
6. Bake for 30 minutes until lightly browned and bubbly. Serve warm or chilled with a dollop of chilled coconut cream.

Variations:

Frozen Berry Option: If using frozen berries, thaw and drain well. Keep in mind that thawed berries will compress, so measure out 8 cups before thawing.

Blueberry Option: If using only blueberries, substitute Frontier Alcohol Free Lemon Flavor throughout the recipe for the Frontier Alcohol Free Orange flavor.

Tip: Fresh raspberries are very delicate and care must be taken when cleaning them. Examine each berry and remove any foreign objects. Fill a bowl with cold water and if you have Grapefruit Seed Extract on hand, put in a couple drops. Gently swish berries in the water, and carefully drain berries. Repeat the process. There's no need to rinse the berries in clear water. GSE in this quantity won't taste, plus it has antifungal properties that aid in elimination of mold and yeast.

Pie Crust

Gluten free pie crust can be foolproof—just a tad more fragile to work with without the gluten. If you roll the crust out between plastic wrap, and follow the directions, you'll be thrilled with the results.

A flaky crust requires cold shortening and ice water, mixing the flours into the fat before the fat is absorbed into the flour. If the fat melts before it's in the oven, your pie crust will be crumbly.

It's all right to use a food processor in step 3 and 4 if you simply pulse until the mixture is crumbly; however, it's really better to use a pastry blender because it's "game over" if the dough heats up. When mixing the egg and other liquids into the dough, be certain to mix by hand.

This recipe was adapted from Gluten-free Sugar-free Cooking by Susan O'Brien, copyright 2006, published by Da Capo Press. We offer Ms. O'Brien's awesome recipe with only a few necessary changes. June

Makes: One or two-crust pie

Prep Time: 40 minutes

Bake Time: 8 to 10 minutes

Ingredients:

One-Crust Pie	**Two-Crust Pie**
3/4 cup brown rice flour	1 1/2 cups
1/4 cup potato starch flour (not potato flour)	1/2 cup
2 tablespoons arrowroot starch	1/4 cup
3/4 teaspoon salt	1 1/2 teaspoons
1/2 teaspoon xanthan gum	1 teaspoon

1/4 cup plus 2 tablespoons chilled shortening	3/4 cup

---

1 small egg or 2 tablespoons liquid egg beaters	1 large egg
1 tablespoon fresh lemon juice	2 tablespoons

Kitchen Tools:

Stand mixer or food processor
Measuring cups and spoons
Whisk
Plastic wrap
Rolling pin
Pie pan
Aluminum foil
Citrus juicer
Small bowl

Instructions:

1. Measure out shortening and place in the freezer for a short time or the refrigerator for a longer time to chill well before using. Do not let the shortening freeze.
2. Preheat oven to 375 degrees F (191 degrees C) if prebaking crust. Grease pie pan and set aside.
3. Wash and juice lemon. Measure out the juice and set aside.
4. Measure brown rice flour, potato starch, arrowroot starch, salt, and xanthan gum into the mixer bowl or food processor. Mix well.
5. Add cold shortening to the flour mix and pulse briefly, just until flour and shortening forms beads or, better yet, use a pastry blender. Remove to a bowl if you've used a food processor.
6. In a small bowl, whisk together the egg and lemon juice. Add to the flour mix and stir just until mixture forms into a ball. Mixture must hold together without crumbling but not be sticky. You may need to work a bit of cold water into the dough to get the right consistency. If so, add 1 tablespoon at a time and knead well.
7. Spritz a bit of water on the counter. Cut 1 piece of plastic wrap approximately 18" long. Smooth the plastic wrap over the moistened area. Divide dough in half if making a two-crust pie, and form one half into a ball. Place on the plastic wrap and cover with another piece of plastic wrap the same size.
8. Gently roll out the dough to a uniform consistency the size of your pie pan. Crust should a little thicker than 1/8" and less than 1/4". Remove top piece of plastic wrap and gently pick up rolled out dough and the bottom piece of plastic wrap. Supporting it carefully with your hand, gently flip it into the pie pan and ease the crust into the pan contours. Carefully peel plastic wrap away from the dough. If this is to be a one-crust pie and there is a dough overhang, fold the excess upward onto the lip of the pie pan. Press to incorporate and make a thicker rim for your crust.
9. If prebaking the crust, prick the crust every couple of inches with a fork to encourage the crust not to puff away from the pie pan. Bake for 8 to 10 minutes and fill with a precooked filling.
10. If this is a two-crust pie, continue to roll out the second ball of dough following the same procedure. Fill pie with filling and place second crust on top of the filling. Crimp the edges to seal.
11. Cut small slits in the top crust to allow steam to escape as it bakes. Since gluten-free flours tend to brown faster than gluten flours, cover the edge of the crust with strips of aluminum foil. Remove foil halfway through the baking time.

Holiday Eggnog

As sometimes happens, a failed recipe gave us a whole new dish and a great new delight. When we converted a rich vanilla pudding recipe into gluten free and sugar free, something went wonderfully wrong. The pudding never entirely set but had the consistency and taste of the commercial eggnog I remembered, only available during the holiday season.

Serve this sweet eggnog chilled in small fancy glasses, sprinkled with nutmeg. It is deceptively rich and meant to be sipped for maximum enjoyment. June

Makes: 4 cups
Prep Time: 5 minutes
Cooking Time: 10 minutes
Cooling Time: 2 hours or more

Ingredients:

3 egg yolks

1/2 cup cold rice milk
1/4 cup plus 1 tablespoon cornstarch

---

2 1/2 cups rice milk
1 cup coconut milk
3 tablespoons vegetable glycerine
3/4 teaspoon SweetLeaf English Toffee liquid stevia
1/4 teaspoon salt

---

1 1/2 tablespoons Frontier Non-Alcoholic Vanilla

Kitchen Tools:

2-quart saucepan

Measuring cups and spoons

Whisk or electric hand mixer

Small bowl

Instructions:

1. Place egg yolks in saucepan, and beat until broken down using either a whisk or a handheld mixer.
2. In a small bowl, stir cornstarch into 1/2 cup cold rice milk until dissolved. Add to egg yolks and mix well.
3. Add the remainder of the rice milk, coconut milk, vegetable glycerine, liquid stevia, and salt. Cook over medium heat, stirring constantly, until mixture thickens and bubbles. Boil 1 minute and remove from heat.
4. Stir in vanilla and chill thoroughly. Serve in small glasses, garnished with a sprinkle of nutmeg.

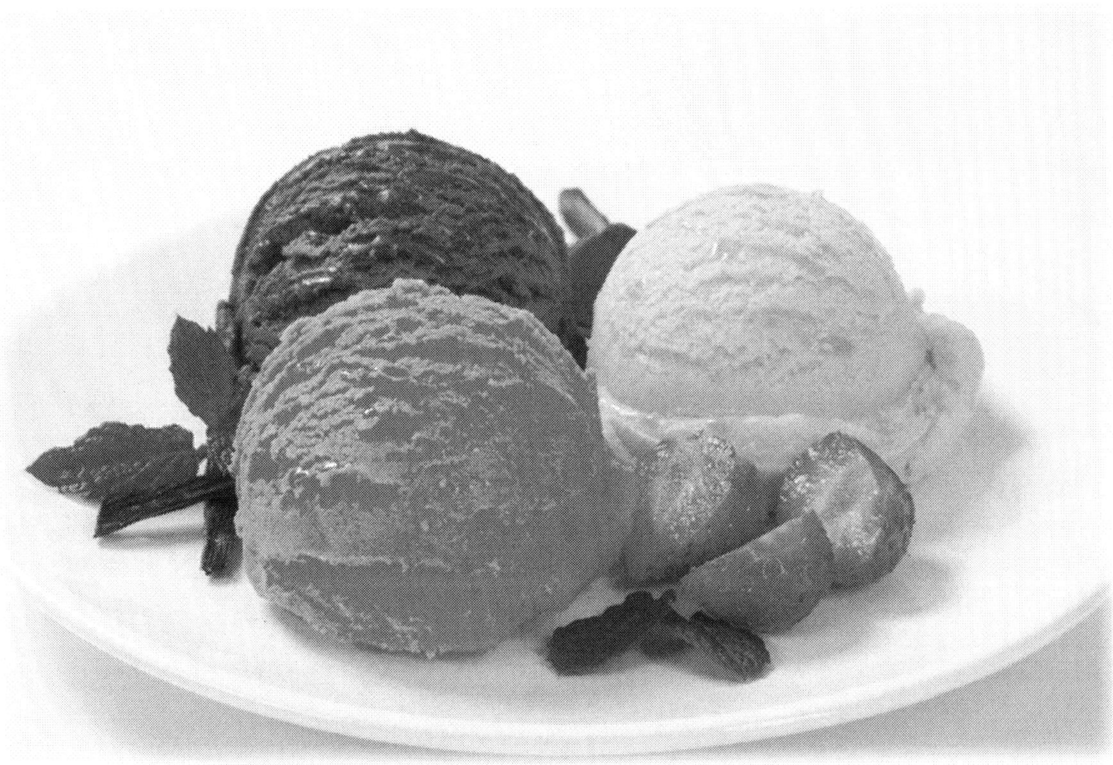

Ice Cream

When we began developing ice cream recipes, it was out of frustration with available commercial ice creams. They all had ingredients Kris and Jonathan could not have, and the challenge was on. Our favorite flavors became the inspiration for each recipe in this section, using only the approved ingredients we could have. All recipes are geared for a small ice cream maker and you'll find the results rich and satisfying.

If you try only one recipe, make it the Chocolate Gelato, which has been compared to authentic Italian gelato. And nothing beats the Velvet Pumpkin Ice Cream at holiday time!

Berry Blast Ice Cream

If eaten in moderation, there are a few berries that do not trigger a Candida-related response in my digestive tract, and a combination of blueberry, blackberry, and raspberry is my favorite. Our first attempts at berry ice creams were bland and uninteresting. Fortunately, we discovered blueberry and cranberry concentrates, and what a difference they made!

Blueberries are a good source of fiber, manganese, and vitamins C and K. They are considered valuable as an anti-oxidant and may contribute to maintaining healthy blood sugar levels as well as help the body fight infections.

The berry flavors blend together beautifully in this dish, and with the addition of the sweetness and subtle taste of the coconut nectar combined with the ice cream base, it's not only esthetically pleasing but a taste-popping delight. Kris

Makes: 6 1/2-cup servings
Prep Time: 35 minutes
Cook Time: 10 minutes
Ice Cream Machine Time: Depends on your machine

Ice Cream Ingredients:

2 large eggs
1 cup rice milk
1 cup canned coconut milk, at least 17g. fat per 1/2 cup
3 tablespoons vegetable glycerine
2 tablespoons coconut nectar
2 tablespoons blueberry concentrate
2 tablespoons cranberry concentrate
2 teaspoons xanthan gum
3/4 teaspoon SweetLeaf Berry liquid stevia
1/4 teaspoon salt

---

1 tablespoon Frontier Non-Alcoholic Vanilla

1/2 cup Berry Blast Sauce

Berry Blast Sauce Ingredients:

1 cup frozen mixed berries, thawed and well drained

---

3 tablespoons berry juice from thawed

1 teaspoon xanthan gum berries

1 teaspoon cornstarch

---

1 tablespoon blueberry concentrate

1 tablespoon water

1 teaspoon coconut nectar

15 drops SweetLeaf Lemon Drop liquid stevia

Kitchen Tools:

1 1/2-quart saucepan

Measuring cups and spoons

Ice cream maker (This recipe is geared toward a small sized machine.)

Blender

Small saucepan

Instructions:

1. Break eggs into blender and add rice milk, coconut milk, vegetable glycerine, coconut nectar, blueberry concentrate, cranberry concentrate, xanthan gum, liquid stevia, and salt. Blend on high for at least 1 minute to dissolve xanthan gum.
2. Pour mixture into saucepan and heat over medium heat, stirring constantly. Bring to a boil.
3. Remove from heat and stir in vanilla. Refrigerate for several hours.
4. Meanwhile, to make the Berry Blast Sauce, drain berries and set aside.
5. In a small saucepan, stir together the berry juice, cornstarch, and xanthan gum until smooth and thick. Add the blueberry concentrate, water, coconut nectar, and liquid stevia. Stir until well combined.
6. Place over medium heat and stirring constantly, boil for 1 minute. Stir in the berries and refrigerate until cool.
7. When the ice cream mixture is thoroughly cooled, pour into ice cream maker and follow manufacturer's directions. When ice cream is properly churned, gently stir in the chilled Berry Blast Sauce. Pour into a freezable container and allow to freeze to a firm consistency.

Chocolate Gelato

Coming from a frugal farming family, when we got ice cream, it was always the cheapest brand of vanilla, with an occasional venture into the exotic when Mom brought home Neapolitan. Although the brand wasn't particularly good, and full of chemicals and artificial flavors, the chocolate portion went first and still evokes sweet childhood memories.

When Kris and I became more conscious of all the foods that triggered reactions in us, we searched through the frozen food sections of many stores to find an ice cream that was dairy free, sugar free, gluten free, and soy free, always coming up empty handed. In desperation, we put our own recipe together from our accepted list of foods, and the end result netted a delightful, wide-eyed smile. We found a winner that tasted very much like rich, smooth gelato. Try it for yourself and you'll agree that you don't miss the sugar or the chemicals! June

Makes: 4 1/2-cup servings
Prep Time: 10 minutes
Cook Time: 10 minutes
Ice Cream Machine Time: Depends on your machine

Ingredients:

2 eggs
1 cup plus 2 tablespoons coconut milk, 14% to 17% fat per 1/2 cup
1 cup rice milk
1/4 cup cocoa powder
3 tablespoons vegetable glycerine
1 teaspoon SweetLeaf Vanilla Creme liquid stevia
1/2 teaspoon xanthan gum
1/8 teaspoon salt

---

2 tablespoons Frontier Non-Alcoholic Vanilla

Kitchen Tools:

Blender

1 1/2-quart saucepan

Measuring cups and spoons

Ice cream maker (This recipe is geared toward a small sized machine.)

Instructions:

1. Break eggs into blender and add coconut milk, rice milk, cocoa powder, vegetable glycerine, liquid stevia, xanthan gum, and salt. Blend on high for at least 30 seconds to dissolve xanthan gum.
2. Transfer mixture to the saucepan and heat over medium heat, stirring constantly. Bring just to a boil but do not allow the mixture to reach a rolling boil. If curdling occurs, pour the hot mixture into a blender and remove the center cover. Place a clean cloth over the cover to allow steam to escape. Start blender on low and then blend on high for at least 30 seconds to reintegrate the texture.
3. Remove from heat and stir in vanilla. Refrigerate for several hours until thoroughly cooled.
4. When mixture is cooled, pour into ice cream maker and follow manufacturer's directions.

Variations:

Chocolate Chip: When ice cream is almost frozen, add 1/4 cup gluten free chocolate chips.

Tip: The history of ice cream is inconclusive, but some sources say ice cream can be traced back to the Chinese in 3000 BC. Early references include the Roman emperor Nero (A.D. 37-68) who ordered ice to be brought from the mountains and combined with nectar, fruit pulp, and honey. By the 1700s, it was being served by George Washington and Thomas Jefferson. Dolly Madison created a sensation when she served ice cream as a dessert in the White House at the second inaugural ball in 1812. In 1843, Nancy Johnson, a New England homemaker, invented the hand-cranked ice cream churn and, in the next thirty years, more than 70 improvements to the original design were patented. In 1983, Cookies 'n Cream became an instant hit, and in 1991, Chocolate Chip Cookie Dough quickly became a flavor phenomenon. Some of the more unusual flavors to be found include Candied Bacon, Garlic (it actually doesn't taste as bad as it sounds), Sauerkraut, Pickle, Avocado, Chili, and Wasabi.

Frozen Chocolate Rice Milk

Many of our recipes use coconut milk because it adds a certain richness in flavor and texture we find most pleasing, but there are times we'd rather not have one more dish that includes coconut. Our goal in this recipe was to eliminate the coconut milk found in our Chocolate Gelato recipe, and still have a "scoop-able" texture along with a satisfying, chocolate taste. While we didn't count the calories, carbs, and fiber in this recipe, we know the Weight Watcher point level is lower when eliminating the coconut milk, yet the flavor and texture is off the chart. We think you're going to love this ice cream! Kris

Makes: 5 1/2-cup servings
Prep Time: 10 minutes
Cook Time: 10 minutes
Ice Cream Machine Time: Depends on your machine

Ingredients:

3 eggs
2 cups rice milk
1/4 cup cocoa powder
3 tablespoons vegetable glycerine
1 teaspoon xanthan gum
1 teaspoon SweetLeaf Vanilla Creme liquid stevia
1/8 teaspoon salt

---

2 tablespoons Frontier Non-Alcoholic Vanilla

Kitchen Tools:

Blender
1 1/2-quart saucepan
Stirring spoon
Measuring cups and spoons
Ice cream maker (This recipe is geared toward a small sized machine.)

Instructions:

1. Break eggs into blender and add rice milk, cocoa powder, vegetable glycerine, xanthan gum, liquid stevia, and salt. Blend on high for at least 30 seconds to dissolve xanthan gum.
2. Transfer mixture to the saucepan and heat over medium heat, stirring constantly. Bring to a boil. If mixture "curdles," return hot mixture to the blender, remove the center cover, place a clean cloth over the cover to allow steam to escape, and blend on high for at least 30 seconds. Remove from heat and stir in vanilla. Refrigerate for several hours until thoroughly cooled.
3. When mixture is cooled, pour into ice cream maker and follow manufacturer's directions.

Variations:

Chocolate Chip: When ice cream has been churned, stir in 1/4 cup gluten free chocolate chips.

Lemon Custard Ice Cream

One of our favorite smells is a fresh cut lemon, which generally draws the other members in the kitchen over the cutting board to inhale deeply. We are always looking for ways to incorporate fresh lemons into our foods, and combining lemon with our love of ice cream resulted in this recipe. We usually have to work with a new recipe a few times to be satisfied with the results, but we got the taste and texture right on the first try.

We think you'll agree that Lemon Custard Ice Cream is a sweet, refreshing dessert that can't be beat on a hot day. Kris

Makes: 4 1/2-cup servings
Prep Time: 10 minutes
Cook Time: 10 minutes
Ice Cream Machine Time: Depends on your machine

Ingredients:

1 tablespoon lemon zest

Juice of 1 lemon

---

2 large eggs
1 cup rice milk
1 cup canned coconut milk, at least 17g. fat per 1/2 cup
1/4 cup vegetable glycerine
3/4 teaspoon SweetLeaf Vanilla Creme liquid stevia
1/2 teaspoon xanthan gum
1/8 teaspoon salt

---

1 tablespoon Frontier Non-Alcoholic Vanilla

Kitchen Tools:

2-quart saucepan

Blender

Measuring cups and spoons

Box grater

Citrus juicer

Ice cream maker (This recipe is geared toward a small sized machine.)

Instructions:

1. Wash lemon and, using the fine side of the grater, make lemon zest. Measure out 1 tablespoon of zest, loosely packed, and set aside.
2. Juice the lemon and add the lemon juice to the blender.
3. Add the eggs, rice milk, coconut milk, vegetable glycerine, liquid stevia, xanthan gum, and salt to the blender. Blend on high for 1 minute to dissolve the xanthan gum.
4. Pour mixture into saucepan and heat over medium heat, stirring constantly until it begins to bubble around the edges. Boil for 15 seconds to facilitate thickening, but not long enough for mixture to curdle. If curdling occurs, pour hot mixture into blender and remove the center cover. Place a clean cloth over the cover to allow steam to escape. Start blender on low and then blend on high for at least 30 seconds to reintegrate the texture.
5. Remove from heat and stir in vanilla and lemon zest. Mixture will be thin. Refrigerate for several hours.
6. When mixture is thoroughly cooled, pour into ice cream maker and follow manufacturer's directions.

Mint Chocolate Chunk Ice Cream

Early in writing this cookbook, upon discovering we could make great tasting ice creams, we thought it would be a snap to make a mint chip ice cream. I should have known better. The "easy" stuff is always difficult. The first problem we encountered was that all chocolate chips had sugars Kris couldn't have. The second issue was when we didn't consider the laws of food chemistry in relation to freezer physics—mint flavor intensifies when frozen. The first batch had so much mint that one taste cleared our sinuses, and the rest deodorized the garbage disposal.

Our final version is a refreshing, cool mint base with sweet chocolate chunks stirred in after the ice cream is churned, perfect with a cup of good English breakfast tea. Kris

Makes: 5 1/2-cup servings

Prep Time: 10 minutes

Cook Time: 10 minutes

Ice Cream Machine Time: Depends on your machine

Ingredients:

2 large eggs

1 cup rice milk

1 cup canned coconut milk, at least 17g. fat per 1/2 cup

1 tablespoon plus 1 teaspoon vegetable glycerine

1 teaspoon SweetLeaf Chocolate liquid stevia

1 1/2 teaspoons xanthan gum

1/4 teaspoon Frontier Alcohol Free Peppermint Flavoring

1/4 teaspoon salt

---

1 tablespoon Frontier Non-Alcoholic Vanilla

1/4 cup leftover chocolate outer coating from Sunbutter Cups (see recipe in Snacks)

Kitchen Tools:

1 1/2-quart saucepan

Blender

Measuring cups

Measuring spoons

Ice cream maker (This recipe is geared toward a small sized machine.)

Instructions:

1. Break eggs into blender and add rice milk, coconut milk, vegetable glycerine, liquid stevia, xanthan gum, peppermint flavoring, and salt. Blend on high for at least 30 seconds to dissolve xanthan gum.
2. Put mixture in saucepan and heat over medium heat, stirring constantly. Bring to a boil. Remove from heat and stir in vanilla.
3. Refrigerate for several hours. When mixture is thoroughly cooled, pour into ice cream maker and follow manufacturer's directions.
4. When ice cream has finished churning, gently stir in the chocolate, which will harden upon contact with the cold ice cream. When incorporated, the chocolate should be in small chunks.

Pebbly Path Ice Cream

It was Sunday morning, and my daughter and grandson were discussing that we needed a new ice cream flavor. I think in a logical sequence of events, come up with a new dish, and then figure out an appropriate name. Kris and Jonathan, on the other hand, are wired differently. They skipped right to the name and then decided what ingredients would fit the name. They wanted to go with the name Rocky Road, but since that was already taken, they decided on Pebbly Path. After brainstorming, we chose a vanilla base with toasted sunflower seeds throughout, and swirls of chocolate and caramel.

The caramel syrup has a base of tapioca syrup, which may not be available in all health food stores or organic markets in your area. It is a light, sweet syrup that has a very low glycemic value, and well worth searching out if you have issues with Candida. Check our list of Product Brands for more information.

The chocolate is leftover chocolate outer coating from the Sunbutter Cups candies. If you make the candy to the proportions described, you will have about half a cup of leftover chocolate. Or you can improvise with something else, if you like. We hope you enjoy the crunch and variations in textures as much as we do. June

Makes: 6 1/2-cup servings
Prep Time: 10 minutes
Cook Time: 10 minutes
Ice Cream Machine Time: Depends on your machine

Base Ingredients:

2 large eggs
1 cup canned coconut milk, at least 17g. fat per 1/2 cup
1 cup rice milk
1 tablespoon vegetable glycerine
1 1/2 teaspoons xanthan gum
1/2 teaspoon SweetLeaf English Toffee liquid stevia
1/8 teaspoon salt

---

1 tablespoon Frontier Non-Alcoholic Vanilla

Swirl Ingredients:

1/4 cup toasted sunflower seeds

1/4 cup tapioca syrup

3/4 teaspoon SweetLeaf English Toffee liquid stevia

1/4 cup leftover chocolate outer coating from Sunbutter Cups (see recipe in Snacks)

Kitchen Tools:

1 1/2-quart saucepan

Blender

Measuring cups and spoons

Ice cream maker (This recipe is geared toward a small sized machine.)

Instructions:

1. Break eggs into blender and add coconut milk, rice milk, vegetable glycerine, xanthan gum, liquid stevia, and salt. Blend on high for at least 30 seconds to dissolve xanthan gum.
2. Pour mixture into saucepan and heat over medium heat, stirring constantly. Bring to a boil.
3. Remove from heat and stir in vanilla. If mixture is not velvet smooth, pour hot mixture into blender and remove the center cover. Place a clean cloth over the cover to allow steam to escape. Start blender on low and then blend on high for at least 30 seconds to reintegrate the texture. Refrigerate for several hours.
4. When mixture is thoroughly cooled, pour into ice cream maker and follow manufacturer's directions.
5. While ice cream is churning, prepare the swirl ingredients. Measure out sunflower seeds and set aside.
6. To make Caramel Syrup, stir together the tapioca syrup and liquid stevia. Set aside.
7. Measure leftover chocolate from outer coating recipe of Sunbutter Cups. Stir to ensure a smooth consistency.
8. When ice cream is properly churned, thoroughly stir in the sunflower seeds and spoon ice cream into a freezer container. Using a back and forth motion, pour caramel syrup and chocolate over ice cream. Using a table knife, cut through ice cream in a back and forth motion to swirl toppings through ice cream. Cover and store in freezer.

Strawberry Ice Cream

After successfully designing seven different recipes for ice cream flavors, I thought making strawberry ice cream would be a snap. In truth, we had some amazing failures in texture and taste that had us scratching our heads, and it proved more complicated than just adding fresh strawberries to the ice cream churn. Early attempts had us microwaving and chiseling ice cream out of the container, and wondering why it didn't taste at all like strawberry.

After a considerable amount of trial and error, we combined the ingredients and process below to give us that fresh taste that "popped." The combination of berry stevia and Valencia orange stevia, as well as the cranberry concentrate, gives this ice cream a rich flavor. If you grow your own strawberries, your ice cream will be even better! June

Makes: 8 1/2-cup servings
Prep Time: 25 minutes
Cook Time: 10 minutes
Ice Cream Machine Time: Depends on your machine

Ingredients:

3 1/2 cups unsweetened frozen strawberries, thawed, mashed, and well drained

---

1 cup strawberry juice from thawed berries
1 teaspoon unflavored gelatin

---

3 large eggs
1 cup canned coconut milk, 17g. fat per 1/2 cup
1/4 cup vegetable glycerine
1 tablespoon arrowroot starch
2 teaspoons xanthan gum
2 teaspoons cranberry concentrate
1 teaspoon SweetLeaf Berry liquid stevia
1/2 teaspoon SweetLeaf Valencia Orange liquid stevia
1/4 teaspoon salt

---

2 tablespoons Frontier Non-Alcoholic Vanilla
1/2 teaspoon Frontier Alcohol-Free Orange Flavoring

Kitchen Tools:

2-quart saucepan

Blender

Measuring cups and spoons

Ice cream maker (This recipe is geared toward a small sized machine.)

Instructions:

1. Thaw strawberries in the microwave in several short sessions and pour off liquid while still cold. Mash and drain strawberries well. You should have about 1 cup of strawberry juice.
2. Stir unflavored gelatin and strawberry juice together in a cup or bowl, and let thicken for a few minutes.
3. Meanwhile, break eggs into a blender and add coconut milk, vegetable glycerine, arrowroot starch, xanthan gum, cranberry concentrate, stevias, and salt. Add the strawberry juice and process on high for 1 minute. Mixture will be thick.
4. Pour mixture into a saucepan. Stirring constantly on medium high heat, heat until thickened and bubbling.
5. Stir strawberries, vanilla, and orange flavoring into mixture and refrigerate for several hours.
6. When mixture is thoroughly cooled, pour into ice cream maker and follow manufacturer's directions.

Vanilla Ice Cream

This recipe came about as a result of our frustration with all brands of conventional ice creams and even the choices in the health food stores. My grandson was almost in tears as he walked through the frozen dessert section of our local grocery store, reading label after label, and putting each container back into the freezer. If you love ice cream, try this recipe the way it is and then get creative. Be sure to email us with your new creation because we love new ideas too. June

Serves: 4 1/2-cup servings
Prep Time: 10 minutes
Cook Time: 10 minutes
Ice Cream Machine Time: Depends on your machine

Ingredients:
2 large eggs
1 cup rice milk
1 cup canned coconut milk, at least 17g. fat per 1/2 cup
1 tablespoon plus 1 teaspoon vegetable glycerine
1 1/2 teaspoons xanthan gum
3/4 teaspoon SweetLeaf English Toffee liquid stevia
1/2 teaspoon SweetLeaf Vanilla Creme liquid stevia
1/4 teaspoon salt

---

2 tablespoons Frontier Non-Alcoholic Vanilla

Kitchen Tools:
1 1/2-quart saucepan
Blender
Measuring cups and spoons
Ice cream maker (This recipe is geared toward a small sized machine.)

Instructions:

1. Break eggs into blender and add rice milk, coconut milk, vegetable glycerine, xanthan gum, liquid stevias, and salt. Blend on high for at least 1 minute to dissolve xanthan gum.
2. Put mixture in saucepan and heat over medium heat, stirring constantly until it begins to bubble around the edges.
3. Remove from heat and stir in vanilla. If mixture is not velvet smooth, pour hot mixture into blender and remove the center cover. Place a clean cloth over the cover to allow steam to escape. Start blender on low and then blend on high for at least 30 seconds to reintegrate the texture. Refrigerate for several hours.
4. When mixture is thoroughly cooled, pour into ice cream maker and follow manufacturer's directions.

Tip: If your ingredients do not have a high enough fat content, your ice cream will be rock hard in your freezer the next day. The taste will be missing a richness, and you'll get a workout scooping it out of the container. You may want to have a second person standing nearby to catch the pieces that flip out of control off your scoop.

Velvet Pumpkin Ice Cream

It has become an early Saturday morning ritual for us to make ice cream, often two different flavors which usually fail to last us a week. This recipe came about after some brainstorming on new flavor possibilities. Kris especially thinks outside the box, while I frequently struggle just to find the box. We eliminated two ideas right off the bat, avocado flavor and butternut squash flavor, and settled on a simple pumpkin flavor.

In order to get enough of the wonderful, rich pumpkin taste, we used a cup of pumpkin puree to 1 and 1/4 cups of coconut milk. To get just the right combination of sweetness, we used coconut sugar, which has a low glycemic index, vegetable glycerine, English Toffee liquid stevia and lucuma powder, all of which can be found in natural food stores or organic markets. The combination of spices and flavors result in a smooth, sweet, satisfying ice cream that is kid approved. June

Makes: 5 1/2-cup servings
Prep Time: 10 minutes
Cook Time: 10 minutes
Ice Cream Machine Time: Depends on your machine

Ingredients:

2 eggs
1 1/4 cups canned coconut milk, at least 17g. fat per 1/2 cup
1 cup pumpkin puree
2 tablespoons coconut sugar
1 tablespoon lucuma powder
1 tablespoon vegetable glycerine
1 tablespoon xanthan gum
3/4 teaspoon SweetLeaf English Toffee liquid stevia
1/2 teaspoon ground cinnamon
1/2 teaspoon ground nutmeg
1/8 teaspoon salt
1/8 teaspoon allspice

---

1 tablespoon Frontier Non-Alcoholic Vanilla

Kitchen Tools:

1 1/2-quart saucepan

Blender

Measuring cups and spoons

Ice cream maker (This recipe is geared toward a small sized machine.)

Instructions:

1. Break eggs into a blender and add coconut milk, pumpkin, coconut sugar, lucuma powder, vegetable glycerine, xanthan gum, liquid stevia, cinnamon, nutmeg, salt, and allspice. Blend on high for at least 1 minute to dissolve the xanthan gum. Mixture will be thick.
2. Pour into saucepan, and stirring constantly over medium heat, bring to a boil. Remove from heat and stir in vanilla. Refrigerate several hours until thoroughly cooled.
3. Pour into ice cream maker and let it do what it does best until desired consistency is reached.

Variations:

Sweet Potato Ice Cream: Sweet potato puree can be substituted for the pumpkin.

Tip: Lucuma is an exotic Peruvian fruit that has been an honored part of their culture since ancient times. It is often found in celebrations and banquet settings because of its distinct and fragrant flavor, which resembles maple syrup. Lucuma is low in acid, low in sugar, and contains an excellent source of carbohydrates, fiber, vitamins, and minerals. It is especially abundant in beta-carotene, niacin, and iron with significant amounts of calcium and phosphorus. One tree can produce as many as five hundred fruits during a year, and lucuma literally becomes the tree of life when field crops are out of season or damaged by drought. The Peruvians use lucuma in ice cream, and it is one of their most popular flavors.

Frozen Vanilla Rice Milk

There are times when we want ice cream but don't want coconut milk in our diet. The solution was to come up with a recipe that was made of just rice milk but still had the richness and taste of a really good vanilla ice cream. This proved more difficult than we had expected, and it took several tries before we got the consistency and taste we wanted. First attempts had us microwaving a rock hard frozen lump until we figured out the proportion of xanthan gum. Try it with your favorite topping or just plain for a sweet treat. Kris

Makes: 4 1/2-cup servings
Prep Time: 10 minutes
Cook Time: 10 minutes
Ice Cream Machine Time: Depends on your machine

Ingredients:
3 large eggs
2 cups rice milk
1 tablespoon plus 1 teaspoon vegetable glycerine
2 1/2 teaspoons xanthan gum
1/2 teaspoon SweetLeaf Vanilla Creme liquid stevia
1/4 teaspoon salt

---

2 tablespoons Frontier Non-Alcoholic Vanilla

Kitchen Tools:
1 1/2-quart saucepan
Blender
Measuring cups and spoons
Ice cream maker (This recipe is geared toward a small sized machine.)

Instructions:

1. Break eggs into blender and add rice milk, vegetable glycerine, xanthan gum, liquid stevia, and salt. Blend on high for 1 minute to dissolve xanthan gum. Mixture will be thick.
2. Put mixture in saucepan and heat over medium heat, stirring constantly. Bring to a boil.
3. Remove from heat and stir in vanilla. If mixture is not velvet smooth, return to the blender. Remove center cover of the blender, place a clean cloth over the opening to allow steam to escape, and process for 30 seconds. Refrigerate for several hours.
4. When mixture is thoroughly cooled, pour into ice cream maker and follow manufacturer's directions.

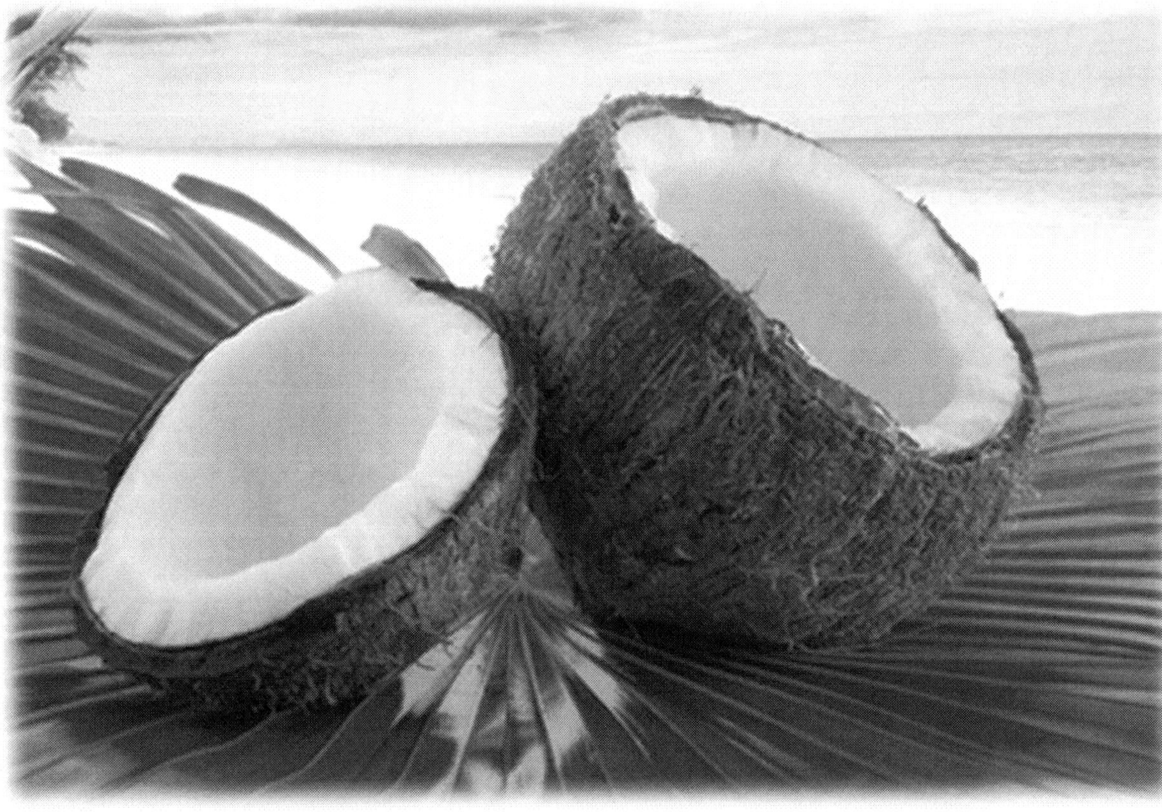

Snacks

Snacks become an important part of a gluten-free diet when dealing with multiple allergies. Especially if you're in the working world, you need something quick if your blood sugar drops or a treat if you're feeling blue. This section has sweet snacks such as candies, granola, and seed butters, as well as homemade crackers that can be dipped in hummus for a pick-me-up or a quick meal.

All snacks in this section are healthy, as long as they are a small part of a balanced diet, and you don't over indulge.

Irresistible Granola

Mom and I had been kicking around the idea of putting together a granola recipe for a couple years, and the only thing that hindered us, was determining how to get the sticky sweetness without honey, sugar, or agave. So we brought out every likely ingredient we had in the pantry and began mixing. Mom knew we had gotten it right when she left the house for a baseball game with my son, before the granola came out of the oven, and when she came back two hours later, half the granola was gone—and I had a guilty look on my face.

This recipe is great as it is, but we urge you to use whatever cereals, seeds, and/or nuts you prefer to make it your own. The only proportions you need to keep in mind are, for the amount of liquids specified, use 5 cups of dry ingredients. Kris

Makes: 5 cups
Prep Time: 35 minutes
Bake Time: 30 minutes

Ingredients:

1/4 cup brown rice syrup
2 tablespoons tapioca syrup
2 tablespoons Frontier Non-Alcoholic Vanilla
3/4 teaspoon SweetLeaf English Toffee liquid stevia
1/4 teaspoon salt

---

1 cup puffed millet
1 cup broken rice cakes
1 cup crispy brown rice cereal
3/4 cup unsweetened coconut flakes
1/2 cup shelled, roasted pumpkin seeds
1/4 cup plus 2 tablespoons sunflower seeds
1/4 cup raw shelled hemp seeds
3 tablespoons golden flax seeds

---

1 cup dried blueberries or any dried fruit your body can tolerate (optional)

Kitchen Tools:

Large baking sheet

Large bowl

Small saucepan

Parchment paper

Instructions:

1. Preheat oven to 250 degrees F (121 degrees C). Cover a large baking sheet with parchment paper and set aside. Oil a large bowl.
2. Heat the brown rice syrup, tapioca syrup, vanilla, liquid stevia, and salt over medium low heat to boiling. Do not microwave, as tapioca syrup and the microwave do not love each other.
3. Mix the puffed millet, broken rice cakes, brown rice cereal, coconut flakes, pumpkin seeds, sunflower seeds, hemp seeds, and flax seeds together in a large bowl. Pour the syrup mixture over the cereals, and stir to coat thoroughly.
4. Spread mixture evenly onto baking sheet, and bake for 30 minutes.
5. Remove granola from oven, pour into a large bowl, and stir in the dried fruit. Allow the granola to cool and enjoy as a snack, over ice cream, or pour cold coconut milk over the granola for a great breakfast. Store in a covered container.

Variations:

Cinnamon Granola: Add 1 teaspoon ground cinnamon to the syrup mixture.

Chocolate Granola: Add 1/4 cup cocoa powder to the syrup mixture as it heats.

Mochi

If you've never had Mochi (pronounced MOW chee), you're in for an interesting treat! Mochi is a gluten free, dairy free, sugar free Japanese food made from a special short-grain sweet rice, that is steamed and pounded to bring out the chewiness and flavor. It is then compressed into a solid sheet. You must have a long, sharp, heavy knife (chef's knife) to cut it into 1" squares, and upon baking, it puffs up into a light, chewy treat.

You will probably not find Mochi at your grocery store, but your favorite health food store should have it in the refrigerated section. If not, ask them to order it. We have tried plain Mochi but prefer the subtle flavor of raisin and cinnamon Mochi. It is best served warm, dipped in a combination of melted, buttery spread, and a sweet syrup of your choice. June

Serves: 4
Prep Time: 5 minutes
Bake Time: 8 minutes

Ingredients:

1 package Raisin & Cinnamon Mochi

---

2 tablespoons buttery spread, melted
3 tablespoons tapioca syrup
1 teaspoon Frontier Non-Alcoholic Vanilla
3 drops SweetLeaf English Toffee liquid stevia

Kitchen Tools:

Cutting board
Long, sharp, heavy knife
Large baking sheet
Parchment paper
Small ramekins

Instructions:

1. Preheat oven to 450 degrees F (232 degrees C). Cover the baking sheet with parchment paper and set aside.
2. Unwrap Mochi and place on a secure cutting board. Mochi is highly compressed and will offer resistance, so take your time in cutting. Using a long, sharp, heavy knife and a rocking motion, cut Mochi into uniform 1 to 1 1/2" pieces.
3. Position pieces on the baking sheet as far apart as possible, as Mochi will puff up and expand. Bake 8 to 10 minutes, checking at the 8 minute mark.
4. While Mochi is baking, melt buttery spread and combine with tapioca syrup, vanilla, and stevia. Pour into individual ramekins.
5. Remove Mochi from oven when it is puffed and brown. Serve immediately with the buttery syrup for dipping.
6. Any leftover Mochi should be wrapped in plastic wrap and used within 2 days.

Perfect Sunbutter

In the beginning of this journey to better health, my frustration level elevated as I discovered each new food allergy, which in effect eliminated almost every prepackaged food. It was especially difficult for me to pack food for work if we didn't have leftovers from the night before. I had always loved peanut butter, but when I developed the allergy to peanuts, sunbutter proved to be an excellent, high-protein substitute. Unfortunately, every brand we found had sugar or some form of sweetener I could not have. The need to make seed butters prompted our purchase of the Bosch Universal Plus mixer and food processor with its powerful motor.

Getting the consistency and taste just right took more experimentation than expected, which meant we ate several batches of less than perfect sunbutter. After trying everything from heating (which made it separate) to adding xanthan gum (which made it slippery), we discovered the solution was in the processing time and strength of the motor. I am unsure if there's any other food processor out there that will grind seeds like the Bosch, so our directions are only geared toward what we know. If you do have a different powerful brand that will work for this, we've described each stage and how the seed butter should look or act. It is the heat caused by the friction of grinding the seeds at a high speed for several minutes, that makes this seed butter smooth and creamy.

We named this recipe Perfect Sunbuttter, because it truly is a perfect blend of sweetness, saltiness, and smoothness without sugar or other unwanted ingredients. Kris

Makes: A little less than 1 cup

Prep Time: 10 to 15 minutes

Ingredients:

1 cup roasted sunflower seeds

---

2 tablespoons plus 2 teaspoons vegetable glycerine

2 tablespoons sunflower oil

1 tablespoon Frontier Non-Alcoholic Vanilla

1/4 plus 1/8 teaspoon salt

7 drops SweetLeaf liquid stevia

Kitchen Tools:

Bosch food processor

Measuring cup and spoons

Rubber scraper

Instructions:

1. Measure sunflower seeds into the food processor, and run on setting 3 or medium to high for 3 minutes, occasionally stopping to push the seeds to the center. The powdery meal will begin to clump as the oils are released from the seeds.
2. Add remaining ingredients into the seeds, and run the processor on high for 2 minutes. The sunbutter should be slightly warm from the friction of processing, somewhat smooth like the consistency of a creamy peanut butter, yet have very small bits of sunflower seeds. You should be able to taste the contrast of the salt and the sweetness at the same time.
3. Cover and store in the refrigerator. If oil separates from the sunbutter, stir before use.

Note: If making a second batch, wash processor blade and bowl in soap and hot water and dry thoroughly. If you omit this step, the sunflower seeds will not have the action needed to properly grind, and oil will not incorporate into the sunbutter.

Variations:

Crunchy Sunbutter: Before step 1, put 1/4 cup roasted sunflower seeds in a food processor. Pulse until the seeds are of desired consistency or "chunkiness." Stir into prepared sunbutter mixture at the end.

Pseudo Saltines

One of the foods we really missed when we went gluten free was saltine crackers. The salty crunch, the way they tasted in soups, and even the way they melted in the mouth were fond memories. We tried a few cracker recipes to rediscover that taste but, even with alterations, each one fell short of our goal.

As so often happens, an accident gave us exactly what we were seeking. It began with a recipe from glutenfreeliving.com for Chickpea Flour Pappadums, an Indian flatbread without a leavening agent. We did not have chickpea flour on hand, so I used gram flour, thinking it was similar enough. As it turned out, they were not interchangeable, but we immediately recognized that the gram flour was the key to getting the saltine flavor we craved. Gram flour can be purchased at oriental super markets, usually in the Indian section. In most recipes, we use it instead of bean flour. In this recipe, either gram or bean flour will work.

After some experimentation with proportions and adding ingredients, we are thrilled with this combination. June

Makes: Approximately 170 1" crackers
Prep Time: 45 minutes
Bake Time: 5 minutes per baking sheet

Ingredients:

1 cup potato starch
3/4 cup gram or bean flour
1/2 cup tapioca flour
2 1/2 teaspoons salt
1 teaspoon xanthan gum
1/2 teaspoon baking soda
1/4 teaspoon white pepper

1/2 cup water
1/4 cup plus 2 tablespoons canola oil

Kitchen Tools:

Food processor
Measuring cups and spoons
Rolling pin
Pizza cutter
Small spatula
2 or 3 large baking sheets
Plastic wrap
Parchment paper
Water spritzer

Instructions:

1. Preheat oven to 475 degrees F (246 degrees C). Line baking sheets with parchment paper and set aside.
2. Measure potato starch, gram or bean flour, tapioca flour, salt, xanthan gum, baking soda, and pepper into food processor. Process to thoroughly incorporate all ingredients, and break up lumps in the potato starch and gram flour.
3. Measure the water and oil into a cup and, with the processor running on high, add oil combination. Process until dough forms into a ball.
4. Cut a piece of plastic wrap approximately 14" long. Lightly spritz your counter with water and lay the plastic wrap down, smoothing out any wrinkles.
5. Sprinkle a bit of potato starch onto the plastic. Forming the dough into a ball, roll it in the potato starch. Cut the dough into four equal portions and dip each exposed side into the potato starch and set aside.
6. Working with one portion of dough at a time, form into a flattened square or rectangle. Using your rolling pin, gently roll out the dough to a thickness of 1/8". If the dough seems too sticky, sprinkle with a bit of potato starch.
7. Gently make puncture holes with your favorite fork like conventional saltines, and cut dough into 1" squares with a pizza cutter. For uniform squares, run the pizza cutter along the edge of a clean plastic ruler. Using a narrow spatula, place each square on the baking sheet. They can be close together because they will puff up a bit but not expand horizontally.
8. Bake for 5 minutes or until lightly browned on the bottom and slightly puffed. Let cool on a rack, and store cooled crackers in a tightly closed container.

Sunbutter Cups

The inspiration for this recipe originally came from Peanut Butter Cups in Sugar-Free Gluten-Free Baking and Desserts by Kelley E. Keough, copyright 2009, published by Ulysses Press. Her recipe is by far the best peanut butter cup I have ever tasted, commercial or otherwise. Unfortunately, Kris has nut allergies and also could not tolerate the agave in the original recipe. We substituted chocolate for the carob powder, and eliminated the hemp seeds in Ms. Keough's original recipe.

These candies satisfy even the sweetest tooth in sugarholics! We toyed with the idea of naming them One More Please, for reasons that will be obvious once you have one. June

Makes: 24 candies
Prep Time: 40 minutes
Cooling Time: 15 minutes

Outer Coating Ingredients:

3/4 cup coconut oil, melted

---

3 tablespoons vegetable glycerine
1 1/2 teaspoons Frontier Non-Alcoholic Vanilla
1 teaspoon cinnamon
3/4 teaspoon SweetLeaf Vanilla Creme liquid stevia

1/2 cup, plus 2 tablespoons cocoa powder

1/4 cup raw cacao nibs

Filling Ingredients:

1/2 cup Perfect Sunbutter (see recipe in this section)

Kitchen Tools:

Small saucepan

Small bowl

Measuring cups and spoons

Small food processor

Mini muffin pans for 24 candies

Mini muffin papers

Instructions:

1. Line mini muffin pans with paper liners and set aside.
2. In a small saucepan, melt coconut oil on very low heat, or gently melt in the microwave, just until melted but not hot. Pour into a small food processor.
3. Add the vegetable glycerine, vanilla, cinnamon, and liquid stevia. Process until blended. Gradually add the cocoa powder and beat until smooth.
4. Stir in the cacao nibs and set aside. If coconut oil separates, simply refrigerate until mixtures cools enough to congeal. Check every half hour until it reaches a more stable consistency.

Filling Instructions:

5. Measure the sunbutter.
6. To assemble the candy, put a thin layer of chocolate in the bottom of each cup. Place 1/2 teaspoon of sunbutter filling in the center of each paper liner, and gently flatten to cover the bottom. If sunbutter sticks to the bottom of the spoon, dip the spoon in a bit of oil.
7. Carefully spoon a scant tablespoon of chocolate over the top to fill cups about 3/4 full.
8. Place candies in the freezer for at least 15 minutes to set, and then store in a covered container in the freezer.

Note: Save any leftover chocolate coating in your cupboard and pour over ice cream or use in Mint Chocolate Chunk Ice Cream or Pebbly Path Ice Cream (see recipes in Ice Cream).

Chocolate Coconut Candy Balls

I spent a Saturday afternoon in the kitchen, and this is what came out of it. I began with a sunbutter base, and added flavorings and fillers to give it stability, flavor, and nutrition. We love chocolate, and the addition of coconut just makes life sweeter.

The candies are kept in the freezer to maintain their integrity, but you will find them easy to bite into. Unless you over indulge, these candies are guilt free and a wonderful treat when you need a quick pick-me-up. Kris

Makes: 40 candies

Prep Time: 40 minutes

Cooling Time: 1 hour

Rolling Time: 15 minutes

Ingredients:

1/2 cup coconut oil, melted

2 tablespoons coconut flour

1/4 teaspoon salt

1/4 cup plus 2 tablespoons Perfect Sunbutter (see recipe in this section)

1/4 cup vegetable glycerine

1 1/2 teaspoons Frontier Non-Alcoholic Vanilla

1 teaspoon ground cinnamon

1 teaspoon SweetLeaf Vanilla Creme liquid stevia

1/2 cup plus 2 tablespoons cocoa powder

1/4 cup raw cacao nibs

1/4 cup hemp seeds or other favorite seed

1/4 cup unsweetened coconut flakes

2 tablespoons ground flax seeds

1/4 to 1/2 cup unsweetened coconut flakes

Kitchen Tools:

Small saucepan

Small bowl

Measuring cups and spoons

Food processor

Waxed paper

Tray that fits in the freezer

Instructions:

1. Mix coconut flour with coconut oil and salt in a small saucepan before heating.
2. Melt coconut oil on very low heat, stirring constantly to ensure the coconut flour doesn't clump. Heat just until melted but not hot. Pour into food processor.
3. Add the sunbutter and process until smooth.
4. Add the vegetable glycerine, vanilla, cinnamon, and liquid stevia. Beat until blended. Gradually add the cocoa powder and beat until smooth.
5. Transfer to a small bowl and stir in the cacao nibs, hemp seeds, 1/4 cup coconut flakes, and ground flax seeds. Refrigerate for 1 hour.
6. Meanwhile, place waxed paper over the tray. You'll want the coconut balls single layer until frozen.
7. Place 1/4 cup coconut flakes in a small, shallow bowl.
8. Mixture will be too sticky to roll in your hands, so use two teaspoons. Scoop out a scant teaspoon and put it in the coconut flakes. Using both spoons to form the candy into a ball, roll the mixture in the coconut. Remove to the wax-covered tray, and continue until all chocolate mixture has been rolled in coconut, adding more coconut flakes as needed.
9. Place candy in freezer for 30 minutes or until frozen. Store in covered container in freezer.

Sunflower Seed Crackies

Kris and Jonathan are always looking for pack-and-go foods and it's a challenge to have enough variety to keep both of them happy. We were dissatisfied with the available gluten-free crackers—most had ingredients we couldn't tolerate, or the flavor made me wonder if anyone tasted them before they went to market. More than one box found its way into our food processor to be camouflaged in another dish. If they passed the safe ingredient and taste test, the cost was prohibitive.

The inspiration for this recipe came from the glutenfreeclub.com, a wonderful resource for Celiac and gluten intolerant information, as well as a huge archive of great recipes. We made lots of substitutions and adjusted amounts to give us the consistency and taste for a dense, tasty cracker that can be dipped or spread. Our head food tester, Julia, commented that the texture was more like a cookie, but the taste was pure cracker, thus the name Crackies. June

Makes: Approximately 40 1" x 2" crackies
Prep Time: 25 minutes
Bake Time: 15 to 20 minutes

Ingredients:

1 cup white rice flour
1/4 cup gram or bean flour
1/4 cup toasted sunflower seeds
1 teaspoon Seasoned Salt (see recipe in Mixes)
1/4 teaspoon Baking Powder (see recipe in Mixes)
1/8 teaspoon xanthan gum

1/2 cup coconut milk
1/4 cup grapeseed oil

Kitchen Tools:

Food processor

Measuring cups and spoons

Large nonstick baking sheet

Rolling pin or waxed paper

Instructions:

1. Place rice flour, gram flour, sunflower seeds, seasoned salt, baking powder, and xanthan gum in a food processor, and process on high for about 2 minutes, until sunflower seeds are ground.
2. Add the coconut milk and oil, and continue to process until well mixed and a ball is formed.
3. Option 1 is to roll out dough to ¼" on a floured surface, and refrigerate for at least 1 hour. Option 2, which is less work, is to form into a roll on waxed paper, wrap, twist the ends of the paper, and refrigerate for at least 1 hour or overnight.
4. Preheat oven to 325 degrees F (163 degrees C).
5. If you've chosen Option 1, cut the rolled out dough into cracker shapes and place on a nonstick, ungreased baking sheet. Crackies expand very little, so they can be close together.
6. If you have chosen Option 2, cut the dough into 1/4" slices and place on a nonstick, ungreased baking sheet, close together. Crackies can be flattened if you want a thinner cracker.
7. Bake for 15 to 20 minutes until crackies have a pleasing, slightly browned color. Cool crackies completely before storing in a sealable plastic bag or airtight container.

Variations:

Herb & Onion Crackies: Add 1 tablespoon Mrs. Dash to the flour mixture, and follow remaining directions.

Sweet Pumpkin Seed Butter

There are a variety of nut butters on the shelves of grocery stores, but there are very few seed butters, which can be frustrating if you have true nut allergies.

It has been said that necessity is the mother of invention; however, I would include that frustration is her sister. This recipe was born out of frustration and inspiration. I could not eat any of the nut butters and there was only one seed butter on the market: sunbutter, which usually contained a risk of ingesting soy, nuts, or something else to which my body was sensitive.

Sweet Pumpkin Seed Butter is intended to meet the need for something both quick and nutritious. Consider serving it on celery, rice cakes, crackers, or a muffin. Let your imagination run wild with all of the possibilities! Kris

Makes: 1 cup

Prep Time: 20 minutes

Ingredients:

1 cup Toasted Shelled Pumpkin Seeds (see recipe in this section)

---

2 tablespoons plus 1/2 teaspoon coconut oil, melted

2 tablespoons vegetable glycerine

1 tablespoon Frontier Non-Alcoholic Vanilla

10 drops SweetLeaf Vanilla Creme liquid stevia

1/4 teaspoon salt

---

2 tablespoons unsweetened coconut flakes

Kitchen Tools:

Heavy duty food processor

Measuring cup and spoons

Instructions:

1. If the pumpkin seeds are raw, please follow the instructions for roasting the seeds in this section. Let cool.
2. Place pumpkin seeds in a heavy-duty food processor, and process on high for 2 minutes until the seeds turn gritty and begin to clump on the sides of the bowl. Occasionally push the clumps down to the center.
3. Add the melted coconut oil, vegetable glycerine, vanilla, liquid stevia, and salt. Process on high for 2 minutes until all ingredients blend together.
4. Add the coconut and mix on high for another 30 seconds. The mixture should be slightly warm from the friction of processing and turned from a gritty substance to a smooth butter, the same consistency as a creamy peanut butter. You should be able to taste the contrast of the sweet and salty at the same time.
5. Store covered in the refrigerator.

Toasted Shelled Pumpkin Seeds

One of the health food stores we often visit offers raw pumpkin seeds, which contain Omega 3 and 6 fatty acids, as well as being high in magnesium, zinc, and protein. Although raw pumpkin seeds are healthy, they are also plain and unexciting. We had just successfully toasted sunflower seeds, so we figured toasted pumpkin seeds would also be a tasty addition to our diet. After some research and experimentation, we came up with this process. It was a huge success!

You can eat Toasted Shelled Pumpkin Seeds plain as a quick pick-me-up, on top of salads, in muffins or granola, and in main dishes to increase the protein value of the dish. This is also the basis for the Sweet Pumpkin Seed Butter recipe found in this section. Experiment and find new ways to enjoy this commonly overlooked nutritious food! Kris

Prep Time: As long as it takes for your oven to heat up
Bake Time: 5 to 7 minutes per pan

Ingredients:
Shelled raw pumpkin seeds
Sea salt

Kitchen Tools:
Large nonstick baking sheet with sides

Instructions:

1. Preheat oven to 350 degrees F (177 degrees C).
2. Spread pumpkin seeds in a single layer on baking sheet, and sprinkle with sea salt.
3. Bake 5 to 7 minutes, watching to ensure they don't burn. If you hear the seeds popping, reduce heat by 25 degrees.
4. Cool completely and store in a covered container.

Toasted Shelled Sunflower Seeds

Sunflower seeds are high in protein, vitamin E, Omega-6 fatty acids, folate, phosphorus, copper, manganese, and selenium. One of many protein sources in our diet, they are the closest thing we've found that taste like peanuts without creating an allergic response often experienced by consuming peanuts. Toasting the raw seeds brings out the "nuttiness" of their flavor. Toss toasted sunflower seeds on a salad, add to breads or muffins, sprinkle on top of ice cream for a little extra crunch, grind into seed butter, or eat by the handful for a quick, healthy snack. Kris

Prep Time: As long as it takes for your oven to heat up
Bake Time: 16 minutes per pan

Ingredients:
Raw sunflower seeds, without the shells
Sea salt

Kitchen Tools:
Nonstick large baking sheet with sides

Instructions:

1. Preheat oven to 300 degrees F (149 degrees C)
2. Spread sunflower seeds in a single layer on a baking sheet, and sprinkle with sea salt.
3. Bake for 16 minutes, watching to ensure they don't burn. If you hear the seeds popping, reduce heat by 25 degrees.
4. Cool completely and store in covered container.

Root'er'scotch Soda

In our quest for better health for the entire family, we attempted to provide flavorful alternatives to my grandson to replace his favorite sugar-filled foods and beverages. Root beer was one of his favorite sodas, or, if you are from the Midwest, you'd call it pop. We gave him a cupboard full of ingredients, full license to experiment, and this recipe was the result. Served over ice, it's a refreshing, sweet, sugar free, and guilt-free beverage. He named it Root'er'scotch Soda, short for Root Beer Butterscotch Soda.

We urge you to experiment with combinations of stevia and flavorings, using this recipe as a rough guide for your own creations. Write down what works for you so you can duplicate it. June

Serves: 1

Prep Time: 2 minutes

Ingredients:

1 cup club soda or seltzer water

13 drops SweetLeaf Vanilla Creme liquid stevia

11 drops SweetLeaf Root Beer liquid stevia

3 drops Frontier butterscotch flavoring

Ice

Kitchen Tools:

Tall glass

Long handled spoon

Measuring cup

Instructions:

1. Gently stir together club soda, stevias, and butterscotch flavoring. Add ice and enjoy!

PASTA

Pasta is found in almost every country in the world and can become the base for a wonderful main course. Search out the pastas available in health food stores or online, if necessary, to get the variety you want. Although we have made gluten-free pasta from scratch, we found it to be labor intensive and prefer to purchase pasta whenever possible.

The exception is one of our favorites called Gnocchi, a pasta made from mashed potatoes and a combination of flours. Our recipe is easy and fun to make, especially for children, and is sure to please.

If you choose to make our White Lasagna, you'll see the lasagna is put together with uncooked noodles, which bake in the sauce. This cuts down on prep time and allows the sauce to permeate the noodles in the oven.

Cheesy Tuna Noodle Casserole

The inspiration for this dish came from a desire to add more fish in our diet. This recipe is for people who don't like the taste of tuna, like me. I enjoyed tuna until I was about six months pregnant with my second child. My first-born child, then in her terrible twos, decided to be a picky eater and would eat only banana or tuna sandwiches. Thinking this was a phase she was going through, I proceeded to make tuna sandwich after tuna sandwich.

If you have ever been pregnant, or know someone who has, you will know that certain smells and foods can change a person's life. With each tuna can I opened, I had visions of an open-air seafood market with chilled eyeballs and fins on ice. It was not long before I was holding my breath every time the catch of the day was drained, scraped out of the can, and mashed between two layers of bread. Twenty-two years later, I am just beginning to eat some seafood again. I didn't think I could ever eat tuna again, until my mom made homemade noodles and put them into this sauce.

This is a wonderful, cheesy-tasting recipe that is gentle yet flavorful, and actually makes the tuna taste more like chicken than fish. This definitely passed the kid and the mom test. Kris

Serves: 4
Prep Time: 50 minutes
Bake Time: 30 minutes

Ingredients:

1 tablespoon buttery spread
1 onion, chopped
2 stalks celery, diced

---

2 garlic cloves, minced

1/4 cup buttery spread
3 tablespoons sweet rice flour

---

2 cups rice milk
1 teaspoon Seasoned Salt (see recipe in Mixes)
1/8 teaspoon ground pepper

---

1 1/2 cups Daiya Cheddar Style Shreds cheese

1/2 cup chopped fresh parsley

---

7 oz. can albacore tuna, drained

---

6 oz. gluten-free noodles

---

1 tablespoon buttery spread

1/2 cup gluten free bread crumbs

Kitchen Tools:

8” x 8” baking dish

Small skillet

Measuring cups and spoons

Medium skillet

1 1/2-quart saucepan

Instructions:

1. Preheat oven to 350 degrees F (177 degrees C). Oil the baking dish and set aside.
2. Heat 1 tablespoon buttery spread in a medium skillet, and add the onion and celery. Stir and sauté until onion and celery are soft. Add the garlic and cook for 1 minute longer. Remove from heat and set aside.
3. To make the sauce, heat 1/4 cup buttery spread in a saucepan until bubbly. Stir the sweet rice flour into the butter, and stirring constantly, cook over medium low heat for 2 minutes.
4. Gradually stir in the rice milk, seasoned salt, and pepper. Continue to cook and stir for 1 minute longer. Add Daiya cheese and cook until melted. Stir in the chopped parsley and sautéed vegetables.
5. Cook pasta according to package directions, just until al dente, drain, and spread in the baking dish.
6. Sprinkle the tuna evenly over the noodles, and pour sauce over the tuna.
7. To make the buttered bread crumbs, heat 1 tablespoon buttery spread in a small skillet over medium or medium low heat. Add bread crumbs, stir, and gently brown for a couple of minutes. Sprinkle crumbs over casserole and bake for 30 minutes.

Gnocchi

Gnocchi (pronounced NYAW' kee) is an Italian pasta made of mashed potatoes, eggs, and flours. Most commercial gnocchi (if you can find a gluten-free brand) are heavy and pasty, but gnocchi are supposed to be light and gently flavorful, lending themselves to sauces or your favorite buttery spread and fresh parsley.

I originally found a recipe at www.celiac.com, a great resource for gluten free living, cookbooks, restaurant guide, recipes, Celiac Disease books, gluten-free products, and so much more. We adjusted some of the ingredients to make this recipe more to our liking.

Traditional gnocchi have ridges to hold the sauce and is achieved by rolling the dough against the tines of a fork. While making your own gnocchi takes a bit of time, they cook up in a couple minutes and you can get your children involved in a fun cooking adventure. The results are stunning! June

Serves: 4
Prep Time: 1 hour 25 minutes
Cook Time: 2 to 3 minutes per batch or 25 minutes total

Ingredients:

2 lbs. cooked mashed potatoes (approximately 4 cups)

---

1 1/2 cups white rice flour
3/4 cup potato starch
1/4 cup cornstarch
1 tablespoon buttery spread
1 tablespoon Daiya Mozzarella Style Shreds cheese (optional)
2 teaspoons salt

---

2 eggs

---

2 quarts or more of boiling water
1 teaspoon salt

Kitchen Tools:

Stand mixer with dough hooks
Measuring cups and spoons
Medium saucepan
Medium to large pot for cooking gnocchi
Potato peeler
Food scale
1 or 2 trays or baking sheets
Waxed paper

Instructions:

1. Line two trays or baking sheets with waxed paper and set aside.
2. Weigh out potatoes, if necessary, then peel, cut into chunks, and place in a medium saucepan. Add just enough cold water to barely cover potatoes, and boil until tender, but not overcooked.
3. Drain potatoes and mash until smooth. Place in stand mixer with dough hooks and allow to cool a bit.
4. Add rice flour, potato starch, cornstarch, buttery spread, Daiya cheese, and salt. Break eggs into opposite side of bowl away from potatoes if they're still hot. Turn mixer on high and beat until well mixed, but don't overbeat. If you prefer, you can refrigerate dough for a couple hours or you can work with the dough if it's still warm.
5. Lightly flour a flat surface with rice flour. Taking small portions of dough no more than 1/3 cup, and using a light hand, roll into a rope about 3/4" thick. If dough is too sticky to work with, add a little more rice flour and gently knead. Cut into 3/4" pieces. Using your favorite fork, gently roll each piece of dough against the tines to make ridges and set aside in a single layer on a tray lined with waxed paper.
6. Heat salted water until boiling in a medium to large saucepan or wok.
7. Gently place a couple dozen gnocchi onto a piece of waxed paper, and ease the gnocchi into the boiling water. They will sink, but in a minute or two will rise to the top. Continue to cook for 2 minutes longer. Remove them with a slotted spoon to a warm, oiled platter in a single layer. To serve, toss with melted buttery spread or olive oil, and add fresh chopped parsley or your favorite sauce.

Note: Cooked gnocchi can be successfully microwaved.
Note: To freeze gnocchi, place uncooked gnocchi in a single layer in the freezer until frozen. Remove and transfer to a covered container or resealable freezer bag. Cook frozen gnocchi 1 1/2 to 3 minutes.

Variations:

Pan Fried: Instead of boiling gnocchi, heat a large skillet with buttery spread and pan fry until slightly browned. Or pan fry after they're boiled for a different taste.

Linguini Alfredo

True Alfredo has been dubbed "heart attack on a plate" due to all the butter, cheese, and cream in the sauce. This version has none of the bad stuff but a wonderful, gentle flavor, an illusion of richness in the sauce, and made of much healthier ingredients. The various vegetables add color, texture, and flavor. This dish is a whole meal in itself, but even more excellent if served with an asparagus side dish. Kris

Serves: 4
Prep Time: 25 minutes
Cook Time: 25 minutes

Ingredients:

2 tablespoons oil

---

2 cups fresh broccoli flowerets, cut into uniform pieces
1 1/2 cups fresh cauliflower flowerets, cut into uniform pieces

---

1 cup carrots, thinly sliced
1 bunch scallions, sliced

---

1 cup bell peppers, in 1/4" rings, 2" long
1 small zucchini, halved and sliced
3/4 teaspoon Seasoned Salt (see recipe in Mixes)
1/2 teaspoon black pepper

---

8 oz. gluten-free linguini

Sauce Ingredients:

2 tablespoons oil
1/2 onion, finely chopped

---

1 1/2 cups salt free Chicken Broth (see recipe in Mixes)

---

1 egg
1/2 cup coconut milk
1/2 cup salt free Chicken Broth
1/4 cup cornstarch

1/2 cup Daiya Mozzarella Style Shreds cheese

1/2 teaspoon salt

Pepper to taste

3 tablespoons fresh chopped parsley

Kitchen Tools:

Nonstick skillet

1 1/2-quart saucepan

Measuring cups and spoons

Whisk or handheld mixer

Small bowl

Instructions:

1. Heat oil in the skillet and add the broccoli and cauliflower. Stir and cook over medium heat for 3 minutes.
2. Add carrots and scallions, and continue to cook for 3 minutes. If broccoli is almost done at this point, remove it and add it back in at the end.
3. Stir in the colored peppers, zucchini, seasoned salt, and pepper. Continue to stir and cook until all vegetables are cooked and broccoli is bright green, approximately 4 minutes. Turn off heat but keep warm.
4. While making the sauce, cook the pasta according to package directions just until al dente and drain.

Sauce Instructions:

5. In a saucepan, heat oil and gently sauté onion until soft and translucent.
6. Turn heat up to medium high and stir in chicken broth.
7. In a small bowl, beat egg and combine with coconut milk, 1/2 cup chicken broth, and cornstarch. Stir to dissolve and then stir into onion mixture. Add the Daiya cheese and stir well.
8. Bring to a gentle rolling boil, reduce heat to low, and cook for 3 minutes, stirring occasionally.
9. Stir in salt, pepper, and parsley. Gently combine vegetables, sauce, and pasta. Serve immediately.

One Pot Chicken & Pasta

With the hope of finding a new old treasure, I went through an ancient recipe box Kris had when she was stationed in England. 95% of the recipes weren't convertible to our present way of eating, but one recipe caught my eye because it was a one-pot meal. Using it as a very rough base, we began experimenting with herbs and quantities to get just the taste we wanted. In the end, our dish did not resemble the original recipe at all, but it served as inspiration to reach our goal of putting together a delicious meal in less than an hour. June

Serves: 4
Prep Time: 15 minutes
Cook Time: 35 minutes

Ingredients:

2 tablespoons buttery spread
1 lb. boneless, skinless chicken breasts, cut into 3/4" pieces
1 1/2 cups onion, chopped
2 cups carrots, sliced 1/8" thick
1 cup celery, sliced 1/4" thick

---

3 cups salt free Chicken Broth (see recipe in Mixes)
2 teaspoons Mrs. Dash Grilling Blends Chicken flavor
1 teaspoon Seasoned Salt (see recipe in Mixes)
1 teaspoon onion powder
1/2 teaspoon paprika
1/2 teaspoon rubbed sage
1/2 teaspoon dried basil
1/2 teaspoon poultry seasoning
1/2 teaspoon garlic powder
1/4 teaspoon black pepper

---

4 oz. uncooked gluten-free pasta

3/4 cup rice milk

1/4 cup plus 2 tablespoons cornstarch

1/4 cup fresh parsley, chopped

Kitchen Tools:

5-quart saucepan

Measuring cups and spoons

Cutting board

Chef's knife

Instructions:

1. Heat buttery spread in the saucepan and add the chicken, onion, carrots, and celery. Sauté, stirring often for 10 minutes.
2. Add the chicken broth, Mrs. Dash, seasoned salt, onion powder, paprika, sage, basil, poultry seasoning, garlic powder, and pepper. Bring to a boil and add the pasta. Stir well to incorporate pasta, cover, and cook according to package directions.
3. Dissolve cornstarch in rice milk and stir into hot mixture. Cook, stirring well until thickened. Stir in parsley and serve.

Roasted Red Pepper Chili Over Pasta

This recipe is designed to give you an alternative to the usual tomato-based chili recipes. For those of us who struggle with Candida, tomato is one of the triggers. Our desire for a dish that was spicy and satisfying, like conventional chili, without the forbidden ingredients, prompted the invention of this recipe.

If you are able to make the red bell pepper sauce in advance, that will greatly cut down on your prep time. If you are making the sauce at the same time, just know this is not a quick dish, but so worth the time and effort. June

–

Makes: 8 cups

Prep Time: 10 minutes

Cook Time: 30 minutes

Time for Red Bell Pepper Sauce: 1 hour 20 minutes

Total Time: 2 hours

Ingredients:

1 lb. lean ground beef

1 large onion, chopped

---

1 15.5-oz. can black beans, drained and rinsed

2/3 cup salt free Beef Broth (see recipe in Mixes)

2 1/4 teaspoons chili powder

2 teaspoons ground cumin

1 teaspoon Seasoned Salt (see recipe in Mixes)

1/2 teaspoon oregano

1/4 teaspoon black pepper

---

1 double recipe Red Bell Pepper Sauce (see recipe in Sauces)

Cooked pasta of your choice

Kitchen Tools:

Large skillet or large saucepan

Measuring cups and spoons

Instructions:

1. Place ground beef and chopped onion in a cold skillet or large saucepan. Using medium heat, brown meat and onion, stirring often.
2. When meat is browned, remove from heat and tip handle upward so fat pools in the pan away from the meat. Spoon fat into a cup and discard.
3. Return meat and onions to medium heat and add the black beans, beef broth, chili powder, cumin, seasoned salt, oregano, and pepper.
4. Stir in a double recipe of Red Bell Pepper Sauce and heat over medium heat until mixture bubbles around the edges. Stirring occasionally, turn temperature to low, and simmer until all flavors incorporate and beans are tender.
5. Meanwhile, cook your favorite gluten-free pasta and drain well. Scoop some pasta into each soup bowl. Top with Chili and serve hot.

Note: If you prefer rice instead of pasta, choose long grain brown rice. The nutty flavor compliments the flavorful Chili perfectly.

Note: Cut down on the time it takes to make this dish by making the Red Bell Pepper Sauce in advance when you have a block of time.

Note: We offer this recipe as an alternative to tomato sauce. If tomatoes aren't an issue for you, substitute your favorite tomato sauce for the Red Bell Pepper Sauce. You may have to adjust the seasonings to your taste.

Roasted Vegetables & Pasta

For 19 years, I was a live-alone happy vegetarian, loving the food, very healthy because of it, and then I moved in with my daughter, son-in-law, and 6-year-old grandson. They were not vegetarian and, for a time, I was cooking two meals every night: one for a vegetarian and one for three omnivores. We quickly figured out that wasn't going to work long term, and at that point, I was ready to join the meat-eating world once again. However, that didn't mean I had to shelve all my great recipes and cookbooks. My favorite vegetarian cookbook is still Weight Watchers' Versatile Vegetarian. It has no weird ingredients, and each recipe is colorful and full of flavor.

There are times when we opt for a meal without meat, and this is one of our favorites. The flavors meld together and yet retain their individual qualities. It's an easy, tasty way to add more vegetables to your diet. We think you'll love the presentation and the flavor, served over your favorite gluten-free pasta. June

Serves: 4
Prep Time: 45 minutes
Roasting Time: 40 minutes

Ingredients:

2 red onions, halved and slivered
1 red bell pepper, seeded, halved and cut into 1/2" strips
1 yellow pepper, seeded, halved and cut into 1/2" strips
1 orange pepper, seeded, halved and cut into 1/2" strips
1 medium zucchini, halved lengthwise and sliced in 1/2" pieces
1 white or Japanese eggplant, cut in 3/4" cubes (optional)
15 garlic cloves, slivered
1/2 cup grapeseed oil
1 1/2 teaspoons Seasoned Salt (see recipe in Mixes)
1/2 teaspoon ground pepper

1/4 cup fresh basil, washed, leaves rolled together and slivered
Daiya Mozzarella Style Shreds cheese

3/4 lb. cooked gluten-free pasta

Kitchen Tools:

Large roasting pan or baking sheet with sides

Your favorite cutting board and sharp knife

Chan or large spoon for turning vegetables

Large bowl

Measuring cup and spoon

Instructions:

1. Preheat oven to 400 degrees F (204 degrees C).
2. In large bowl, combine the vegetables, grapeseed oil, seasoned salt, and ground pepper. Toss to coat and spread in baking pan.
3. Roast for 40 minutes or until all vegetables are soft, turning them every 15 minutes to promote even roasting. If necessary, turn roasting pan 180 degrees if your oven does not heat evenly.
4. Remove from oven, stir in the basil, and serve over your favorite cooked pasta. Top with Daiya cheese.

Variations:

Asparagus Option: Replace eggplant with 1 lb. asparagus. Rinse asparagus, snap off tough ends, and cut into 2” lengths.

White Lasagna

As Kris discovered more and more foods her body wouldn't tolerate, many of our favorite dishes were eliminated, and lasagna was one of those foods we very much missed. Without tomato sauce, ricotta cheese, and mozzarella, it was difficult to imagine lasagna. Much of our new diet required us to think outside the box and White Lasagna is the result of such thinking.

Finding lasagna noodles proved to be no easy task, but we discovered DeBoles Gluten-Free Rice Lasagna Noodles in a local natural food store. If you can't find lasagna noodles, you might try making them yourself if you have a pasta maker. Another option is to search the internet for pasta.

This lasagna is put together with uncooked noodles, which become tender in the oven. The flavorful cream sauce, cooked chicken, layer of sautéed vegetables, and Daiya Mozzarella Style Shreds on top, provide a wonderfully satisfying meal that is kid approved. June

Serves: 6 (you'll want large servings)
Prep Time: 1 hour 25 minutes
Bake Time: 65 minutes
Rest Time: 5 minutes

Ingredients:

1 10-oz. box DeBoles Gluten Free Rice Lasagna Noodles

---

2 tablespoons oil
1 lb. chicken cutlets or breasts, cut in 1" pieces
1 large onion, chopped
1 teaspoon non-salt seasoning such as Mrs. Dash
1/2 teaspoon Seasoned Salt (see recipe in Mixes)

---

1 red bell pepper, diced

---

1 medium zucchini, quartered lengthwise and sliced thin

---

4 garlic cloves, minced

Sauce Ingredients:

2 tablespoons oil

1 onion, chopped

---

3 cups salt free Chicken Broth (see recipe in Mixes)

---

2 eggs

3/4 cup coconut milk

3/4 cup cold salt free Chicken Broth

1/4 cup plus 2 tablespoons cornstarch

2 1/4 teaspoons sea salt

1/2 teaspoon white pepper

3/4 cup chopped parsley

1 cup Daiya Mozzarella Style Shreds cheese

Kitchen Tools:

Small bowl

Medium skillet

Measuring cups and spoons

Whisk

Lasagna pan

2 1/2-quart saucepan

Aluminum foil

Instructions:

1. Preheat oven to 350 degrees F (177 degrees C). Oil lasagna pan and set aside.
2. Heat oil in skillet over medium high heat and add chicken, chopped onion, non-salt seasoning, and seasoned salt. Sauté, stirring often, for 5 minutes.
3. Add diced bell pepper and sauté for 3 minutes.
4. Add zucchini and sauté for another 5 minutes until vegetables are tender.
5. Stir in garlic and cook for 1 minute. Remove from heat but keep warm.
6. To make cream sauce, heat 2 tablespoons oil in a saucepan and add the chopped onion. Sauté, stirring often, until onion is translucent and soft. Add 3 cups chicken broth and heat.
7. In a small bowl, whisk eggs, coconut milk, 3/4 cup cold chicken broth, cornstarch, sea salt, and white pepper. Mix well and stir into onion mixture. Heat and stir until bubbling and thickened. Stir in chopped parsley.
8. To construct lasagna, do not boil noodles, as they will cook in the oven.
    - Spread a cup of sauce in the bottom of the lasagna pan.
    - Place a layer of uncooked noodles on the sauce.
    - Spread 1/4 of sauce over the noodles.
    - Spread all the vegetables and chicken over sauce.
    - Add a layer of noodles.
    - Spread 1/4 of sauce over noodles.
    - Add another layer of noodles.
    - Top with the remainder of the sauce and ensure all noodles are covered.
9. Cover pan tightly with foil and bake for 55 minutes.
10. Remove from oven and sprinkle top of lasagna with Daiya cheese. Return to oven uncovered, and bake for 10 minutes or until cheese melts. Remove from oven and allow lasagna to rest for 5 minutes before serving.

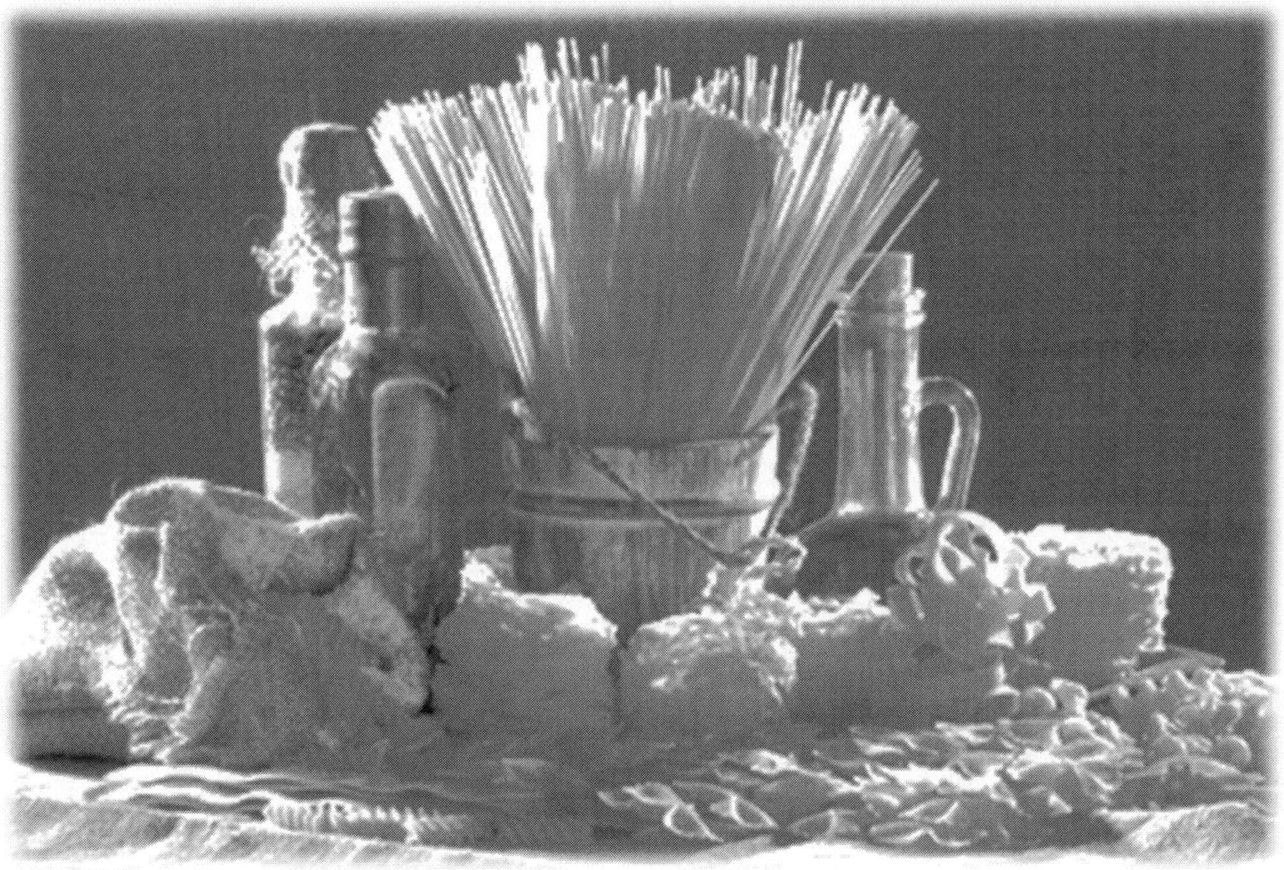

Pasta & Spinach

This dish is not only beautiful, but also flavorful and quick to make. The original recipe was shared at a Weight Watcher meeting in Leominster, Massachusetts, and geared toward a low points single serving. We've expanded on it, but kept the original intent of good nutrition with low calorie and low fat content.

The best pasta is any type that has ridges or curly texture to hold the spinach and flavors. Choose what appeals to you the most, and cook only until al dente so it holds up well when combined with the spinach. June

Serves: 4 as a side dish or 2 to 3 as vegetarian main course

Prep Time: 5 minutes

Cook Time: 30 minutes

Ingredients:

8 oz. ridged pasta of your choice

---

2 tablespoons oil

4 garlic cloves, minced

---

1 lb. fresh spinach, chopped

1 cup salt free Chicken Broth (see recipe in Mixes)

3/4 teaspoon Seasoned Salt (see recipe in Mixes)

1/2 cup Daiya Mozzarella Style Shreds (optional)

Kitchen Tools:

Large skillet

Measuring cup and spoons

Saucepan to cook pasta

Instructions:

1. Heat salted water in saucepan to boiling, and add the pasta of your choice. Cook just until al dente and drain well.
2. While pasta is cooking, gently heat oil on medium low heat in a large skillet. Add garlic, stir and cook for no longer than 1 minute or the garlic will become bitter.
3. Add the spinach, chicken broth, and seasoned salt. Increase heat to medium high. Cover and steam spinach until tender or about 5 minutes. Stir occasionally to incorporate salt.
4. Add cooked pasta and toss to mix well. If there's too much liquid, continue to heat over fairly high heat for a bit, to reduce liquid and intensify flavors. If using Daiya cheese, sprinkle over individual servings and microwave to melt.

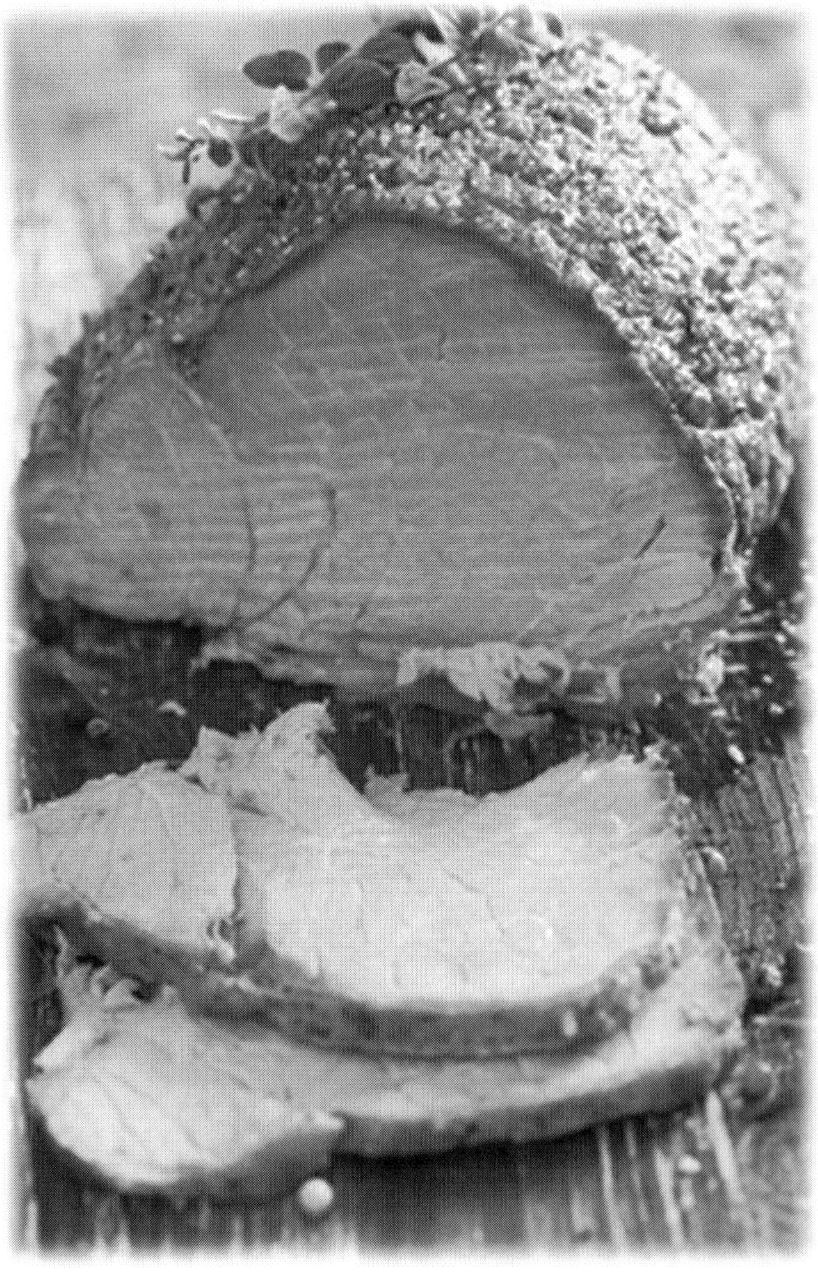

Beef

Growing up on a family owned dairy farm had some wonderful benefits. We knew exactly where our meat came from, and were confident it had been fed only the most natural feeds. Best of all, we got to eat what we raised. At the time, I didn't realize how delicious home raised beef was, and it wasn't until years later, I learned how different commercially raised beef tasted. If you can afford to purchase grain fed, organic beef, you will notice a difference.

This section contains dishes with a variety of preparation and cooking methods, including marinating, baking, stove top, and crock pot cooking. Many of the dishes are comfort foods and all are deliciously flavorful and designed to delight.

Flank Steak Italian Style

This recipe is an adaptation of a recipe found on www.myspicesage.com. We discovered this website when we were searching for particular herbs we couldn't find at the grocery store and felt like we had stumbled into spice heaven. Check out their website and you will quickly see that there's a wealth of information about each herb, including other common names, the taste or aroma category, and substitutions.

The multitude of dried herbs in this recipe gives the flank steak a wonderful, rich flavor. It requires marinating for at least an hour, but is much better if you allow 8 to 18 hours. Flank steak, which tends to be tough, is sliced against the grain on a bias to give you wider slices. This dish is pan-fried to allow the marinade to continue to cook into the steak and release all the wonderful flavors with each bite. June

Serves: 4
Prep Time: 20 minutes
Marinating Time: 1 to 18 hours
Cook Time: 20 minutes

Ingredients:

1 1/2 to 2 lbs. flank steak (see note below on how to slice)

---

1 lemon, juiced

---

3 tablespoons olive oil
2 teaspoons garlic powder
1 teaspoon ground thyme or savory
1 teaspoon Seasoned Salt (see recipe in Mixes)
1/2 teaspoon ground rosemary
1/2 teaspoon ground marjoram
1/2 teaspoon oregano
1/2 teaspoon paprika
1/2 teaspoon black pepper

---

3 tablespoons oil
1 large onion, quartered and sliced

Kitchen Tools:

Large bowl

Whisk

Measuring spoons

Citrus juicer

Large skillet

Instructions:

1. For the greatest ease in slicing the beef, wrap steak in plastic wrap and place in your freezer for 45 minutes. Remove from the freezer, discard the plastic wrap, and cut the steak in thin slices by cutting against the grain and on the bias. If you're unsure what that means, lay the steak out on a cutting board and look at the way the grain goes—usually the length of the steak—and position the meat so the grain runs horizontally to you. Cutting on the bias is achieved by placing your knife at a 45-degree angle and slicing across the grain. This will give you wider slices than if your knife was straight up and down, increase the area to be marinated, and will aid in creating more tenderness.
2. Juice lemon and pour into a medium bowl large enough to marinate all the steak. Add the oil, garlic powder, savory, seasoned salt, rosemary, marjoram, oregano, paprika, and pepper. Whisk to mix well and add the steak, stirring to ensure all steak is coated. Cover and refrigerate up to 18 hours.
3. Heat 3 tablespoons oil in a large skillet over medium heat. Add sliced onion to skillet, cooking and stirring for 5 minutes.
4. Turn heat to medium high and pour steak and marinade into skillet. Continue to cook steak and onions together for 15 minutes, stirring occasionally, until onions are translucent and steak is done.
5. Serve hot over rice, if desired.

G'ma's Swedish Meatballs

My Aunt Sylvia has an infectious personality and a permanently up-tilted mouth that graces her sweet face. She always has a ready smile and laughs easily, whether it's at her own expense or humor injected into her stories. An afternoon over coffee and cake in the presence of Aunt Sylvia always left my sides aching from laughing.

Being a farmer all her life in Minnesota, she was always a great cook, accustomed to preparing meals in a bygone era for threshing crews. One of her very excellent recipes was for Swedish Meatballs, an oven-baked dish that produced mouth-watering results. We've taken her recipe and rebuilt it, but maintained her taste standards. The meatballs are pretty true to the original recipe, but the sauce has been altered to eliminate ingredients that cause allergic reactions. The result is a deliciously sauced meatball dish that can be served over mashed potatoes, rice, or your favorite gluten-free pasta. Bon appetite, farm style! June aka G'ma

Serves: Half a threshing crew or 6
Prep Time: 60 minutes
Total Bake Time: 1 hour 30 minutes

Meatball Ingredients:

2 lbs. lean ground beef
1 egg
1 cup gluten free bread crumbs
1/2 cup hot, salt free Beef Broth (see recipe in Mixes)
1/2 cup chopped onions
1 1/2 teaspoons Seasoned Salt (see recipe in Mixes)
1/2 teaspoon pepper

Sauce Ingredients:

2 tablespoons oil
1 cup chopped onion

---

2 cups salt free Beef Broth

---

2 eggs
1 cup cold rice milk
1/2 cup coconut milk
1/4 cup arrowroot starch
1 teaspoon Seasoned Salt
1/2 teaspoon pepper
6 garlic cloves, minced

Kitchen Tools:

Medium bowl

Measuring cups and spoons

Large nonstick baking sheet

Oven proof casserole dish (approximately 2 1/2-quart)

2 1/2-quart saucepan

Small mixing bowl

Whisk or handheld mixer

Instructions:

1. Preheat oven to 350 degrees F (177 degrees C). Oil casserole dish and set aside.
2. In a medium bowl, place the ground beef, egg, bread crumbs, beef broth, onions, seasoned salt, and pepper. Mix with your hands until well combined or use your mixer with dough hooks.
3. Form into balls about 1 1/2" in diameter and place in a single layer on a large, nonstick baking sheet. This can be done with your hands or by utilizing a melon baller. Bake for 30 minutes. Remove from oven, pour off and discard any accumulated fat, and place meatballs in casserole dish. They can be layered.
4. Meanwhile, make the sauce by heating the oil in a saucepan and adding the chopped onion. Sauté over medium heat until onions are soft and translucent, stirring often. Add beef broth and continue to heat.
5. In a separate small bowl, combine eggs, rice milk, coconut milk, arrowroot starch, seasoned salt, pepper, and minced garlic. Add to saucepan and, stirring constantly, boil for 1 minute.
6. Pour sauce over meatballs and bake uncovered for 1 hour. Serve over mashed potatoes, rice, your favorite gluten-free pasta, or cooked spaghetti squash.

Roast Beef Italiano Au Jus

This recipe came about because we had three roasts in the freezer and no other beef. It was beef night on our rotation plan and the idea of a pot roast made my taste buds yawn.

The liberal seasonings in this recipe lend themselves well to beef, and the end product is a tasty, tender roast with a delicious au jus sauce. This recipe could easily be converted to the crockpot cooking method, and the taste will be the same. We've given you directions for the stovetop, but feel free to do what works for you. It's a matter of convenience and your preference. June

Serves: 4

Prep Time: 5 minutes

Cook Time: 4 hours

Ingredients:

3 lbs. rump roast

2 tablespoons olive oil

---

1 tablespoon non-salt seasoning, such as Mrs. Dash Table Blend

1 tablespoon Italian seasoning

1 1/2 teaspoons dried oregano

1 1/2 teaspoons dried basil

1/2 teaspoon Seasoned Salt (see recipe in Mixes)

1/2 teaspoon black pepper

---

2 cups salt free Beef Broth (see recipe in Mixes)

4 garlic cloves, minced

Kitchen Tools:

4 1/2-quart saucepan

Small shallow bowl

Garlic press

Instructions:

1. In a shallow bowl, mix the non-salt seasoning, Italian seasoning, oregano, basil, seasoning salt, and pepper.
2. Rub olive oil on all surfaces of the roast and roll the roast in the seasonings. Place meat in the saucepan and add the beef broth and garlic.
3. Heat to boiling, reduce heat to low, cover and cook for 4 hours until meat is fork tender. Turn roast occasionally and ensure liquid does not evaporate.
4. Slice roast and arrange on a platter with a bit of au jus over the top. Serve the rest of the au jus on the side.

Variations:

Pot Roast Italiano Au Jus: Use a slightly larger pan and add carrots cut into 2" chunks, a large onion cut into quarters and then crosswise, and small whole potatoes or larger potatoes cut into pieces about 2" thick. Cook on low for the full 4 hours. If desired, thicken broth after cooking to a gravy consistency.

Shepherd's Pie

I was in my mid 20s, serving in the Air Force and stationed in England. There was a lot of farmland around our base, including one farm that raised and sheared sheep. Every spring, we looked forward to the birth of little lambs and would always drive by the field slower than usual to watch the little ones play.

One evening, our live-in nanny made Shepherd's Pie for us, and I instantly knew I had found a new favorite food! The hamburger with gravy topped with mashed potatoes and cheese appealed to the farm girl in me. The vegetables were just extra goodness and nutrition added to an already awesome meal! Even today, when I think of Shepherd's Pie, I remember my roots in Minnesota, but I also remember those wonderful English days imagining a shepherd's joy and the excitement of exploring new possibilities.

This recipe is very adaptable to whatever you have in the fridge or freezer. You can use frozen veggies to cut down on some of the prep time; although, I don't recommend using broccoli—it gets too mushy. Sliced water chestnuts add a nice crunch. Or you can make it without the vegetables! Have fun and create your own new possibilities! Kris

Serves: 4 (unless you want seconds)
Prep Time: 60 minutes
Bake Time: 35 minutes

Ingredients:

1 1/4 lbs. red bliss potatoes, washed and cut into 1/2" slices

---

1/2 cup rice milk
1 tablespoon buttery spread
1/4 teaspoon Seasoned Salt (see recipe in Mixes)
1/8 teaspoon ground black pepper

---

1 lb. lean ground beef
1 onion, chopped
1/2 teaspoon Seasoned Salt

---

2 garlic cloves, minced

---

1 1/2 cups washed, peeled carrots, cut into 3/8" slices
1 1/2 cups celery, cut into 1/4" slices

3/4 cup salt free Beef Broth or part Vegetable Broth (see recipes in Mixes)
1 teaspoon dried basil
1/2 teaspoon Seasoned Salt
1/8 teaspoon pepper
1/8 teaspoon cayenne pepper

1/2 cup Daiya Cheddar Style Shreds cheese
Paprika

Kitchen Tools:

2 1/2-quart cooking pot
Medium sized skillet
Measuring cups & spoons
11-cup ovenproof casserole dish or 8" x 11" x 1" baking dish

Instructions:

1. Preheat oven to 350 degrees F (177 degrees C) and coat baking dish with oil.
2. Place potatoes in the cooking pot and barely cover with cold water. Bring to a boil and cook for 8 minutes or until fork tender. Drain the potatoes, return them to the pan, and add the rice milk, buttery spread, 1/4 teaspoon seasoned salt, and 1/8 teaspoon pepper. Mash until smooth and set aside, keeping potatoes warm.
3. Heat a nonstick skillet over medium heat and add the ground beef, onion, and seasoned salt. Cook for 5 or 6 minutes, breaking up clumps and stirring occasionally until browned. Add garlic and continue to stir and cook for 1 minute. Shut off heat and tip skillet, propping up the handle end so the fat drains away from the meat. Remove fat, reserve 1 tablespoon and discard the rest. Scoop out the meat and transfer to the prepared casserole dish.
4. Return the skillet to medium high heat with 1 tablespoon of beef fat and add the carrots and celery. Cook for 5 minutes, stirring often until just tender. Add the beef broth, basil, seasoned salt, pepper, remaining 1/2 teaspoon salt, 1/8 teaspoon pepper, and cayenne pepper. Cook for 2 or 3 minutes or until the liquid is almost evaporated.
5. Spread the vegetables evenly over the beef. Top with the mashed potatoes and bake for 25 to 30 minutes, or until the potatoes are lightly browned.
6. Remove casserole from the oven and fire up your broiler. Sprinkle Daiya cheese over the mashed potatoes and sprinkle with paprika. Place under broiler for a few minutes until cheese is slightly browned. Watch closely to prevent Daiya cheese from burning. Let sit for a few minutes before serving.

Tacos Our Way

Tacos are a wonderful way to get more raw vegetables into your diet if you do it right. Unfortunately, taco shells that don't have soybean oil, gluten, or artificial coloring are difficult to find. Then there's the mess factor. I prefer to eat my food and not wear it, but a little bit of creativity will allow you to have a satisfying meal, and get in your servings of vegetables at the same time.

Although cutting fresh vegetables can be time consuming, this is a whole meal in itself and well worth the prep time. It's also an excellent opportunity to get your kids involved in meal preparation. We use the time to communicate on a fun level. June

Serves: 4

Prep Time: 50 minutes

Cook Time: 15 minutes

Ingredients:

1 lb. hamburger

1 small onion, chopped

1/2 cup Vegetable Broth (see recipe in Mixes) or water

2 tablespoons Taco Seasoning (see recipe in Mixes)

Lettuce, shredded

3 scallions, thinly sliced

2 stalks celery, diced

1 cucumber, peeled, seeded and diced

1 carrot, shredded

1 red bell pepper, diced

1 yellow pepper, diced

1 ripe avocado, peeled and sliced

Daiya Pepperjack Style Shreds cheese

Tortilla chips

Kitchen Tools:

10" skillet

Cutting board

Sharp knife

Varying sizes of small serving bowls

Instructions:

1. Prepare vegetables and place each in its own serving bowl.
2. Brown hamburger and onion in a dry skillet over medium to medium high heat. Break up the hamburger as it cooks and keep stirring until browned. Remove from heat. Drain and discard the excess fat.
3. Stir the taco seasoning and water into the meat. Heat over medium or medium low heat, stirring often until excess liquid is evaporated.
4. To assemble your meal, break up tortilla chips on your plate. Layer meat, cheese, and vegetables in any desired order, and eat with knife and fork.

Tip: Avocados are a fruit, not a vegetable. Hass is a common avocado variety and the only one grown year round. It's the one with the dark, nubby shell. If you are using the avocado immediately, select one that yields to gentle pressure on the skin at the large end of the fruit. If you plan to use the avocado in a few days, choose firmer fruit that does not yield to the squeeze test and let them ripen at room temperature for a few days. Avocados are rich with nutrients such as vitamin B6, vitamin E, dietary fiber, vitamin C, potassium, magnesium, and folate, as well as being cholesterol and sodium free. Avocados have 60% more potassium per ounce than bananas.

Foiled Round Eye Roast

This recipe was drawn on memories of a baking method from 40 years ago. I would sprinkle a package of dry Lipton Onion Soup over a roast, seal it in heavy-duty foil, put it in the oven at a very low temperature, and go off to work. When I came home, the house smelled wonderfully of onion and fragrant, moist beef. While the Lipton's Soup mix is a thing of the past because of allergies, the cooking method is still very much alive. I particularly like the fact that this process is designed to be started and then forgotten while I go off and have fun. The flavors and juices are locked within the foil and render the meat tender and flavorful. June

Serves: 6
Prep Time: 10 minutes
Bake Time: 7 to 8 hours

Ingredients:

3 lbs. round eye roast, with any fat removed
1/4 cup Onion Soup & Dip Mix (see recipe in Mixes)
1/2 cup salt free Beef Broth (see recipe in Mixes)

Kitchen Tools:

8" x 11" baking pan
Measuring cup
Heavy duty aluminum foil or double layers of regular foil

Instructions:

1. Preheat oven to 250 degrees F (121 degrees C).
2. Tear off a piece of heavy duty aluminum foil or double regular foil, large enough to wrap loosely around the roast, plus a few extra inches to allow expansion and room for juices. Place roast in the center of the foil and sprinkle with the onion soup mix. Bring long ends of foil up, add beef broth, and fold over at least twice to create a seal. Do the same with each side so the roast is totally sealed.
3. Place in baking pan with sealed edges up and bake for 7 to 8 hours. Unwrap and serve. Roast will be tender and moist.

Hamburger Onion Gravy

Ground beef's versatility makes it one of our favorite meats. Recipes can be complicated or quick and simple, and this recipe falls into the latter category. We whipped a meal together that got rave reviews one evening when we had little time and a pound of ground beef thawed out. The ingredients are few, but the results are tasty and satisfying. Kris

Serves: 4
Prep Time: 5 minutes
Cook Time: 30 minutes

Ingredients:

1 lb. ground beef
1 large onion, chopped
2 teaspoons Seasoned Salt (see recipe in Mixes)

---

2 cups salt free Beef Broth (see recipe in Mixes)
2 teaspoons Mrs. Dash or other non-salt onion and garlic mix

1/2 cup cold water
1/4 cup plus 1 tablespoon Bette Hagman's Featherlight Flour Mix (see recipe in Mixes)

Kitchen Tools:

Nonstick skillet
Cutting board
Chopping knife
Measuring cups and spoons
Cup or small bowl

Instructions:

1. In a skillet on medium high heat, brown the ground beef, onion, and seasoned salt, breaking up the meat as it cooks. When meat is browned and onions are translucent, remove from heat and allow fat to drain away from meat. Spoon off any fat in the pan and discard.
2. Return meat to medium high heat and add the beef broth and non-salt seasoning. Bring to a boil.
3. Measure cold water into a cup or small bowl, and stir in the flour mix until dissolved. Pour mixture into meat and broth, stirring constantly as it heats and thickens. Continue to cook for 1 or 2 minutes, and serve over mashed potatoes or rice.

Sirloin Indian Style

Sirloin is a wonderful cut of beef that lends itself well to a marinade, and Indian spices accentuate its flavor. My love of Indian food began when I was stationed in England. Our favorite restaurant was The Tandoori in Shefford and it became a meeting place for our friends, as well as the perfect place to celebrate special occasions.

Indian spices can be incredibly varied and some are very expensive. Favorite Indian dishes taste as different as each Indian family who makes them, and we are definitely not experts in this cooking genre. Consequently, this recipe has no exotic spices, but the combination in the marinade gives the meat a special flavor when broiled. Enjoy this easy way to put different flavors into your steak meal. Kris

Serves: 6
Prep Time: 15 minutes
Marinating Time: Up to 8 hours
Broil Time: Depends on your preference for doneness

Ingredients:
1 1/2 to 2 lbs. sirloin steak

Juice of 1 lime
4 garlic cloves, minced
1/4 cup salt free Beef Broth (see recipe in Mixes)
1 teaspoon ground cumin
1 teaspoon salt
1/2 teaspoon ground turmeric
1/2 teaspoon ground coriander
1/2 teaspoon ground rosemary
1/2 teaspoon black pepper

Kitchen Tools:

Broiler pan

Covered container for marinating

Measuring spoons

Garlic press

Citrus juicer

Instructions:

1. Cut steak into serving size pieces.
2. Juice lime and mince garlic. Put in container for marinating, along with the remaining ingredients. Combine well and add steak, turning each piece to cover all sides. Cover and refrigerate up to 8 hours.
3. Remove beef from marinade and dispose of leftover marinade. Fire up your broiler and cook meat to desired doneness, taking into consideration the thickness of the meat and distance from broiler.
4. Serve immediately with your favorite side dishes.

Meatloaf

Meatloaf was a favorite in our farm diet when I was a kid. We raised our own grain-fed beef, which tasted much different than what we get from the grocery store today. Part of the allure of meatloaf for me was always the ketchup that was baked on top, and I couldn't imagine meatloaf without it. Since ketchup is a forbidden food for Kris and me, we had to come up with a taste that had the satisfying flavor without tomatoes, vinegar, or sugar. We packed a lot of flavor into this dish and accomplished our goal. June

Serves: 4
Prep Time: 25 minutes
Bake Time: 1 hour to 1 hour 15 minutes

Ingredients:
1 lb. lean ground beef
1/2 cup gluten free bread crumbs
1 egg
1/2 cup salt free Vegetable Broth or Beef Broth (see recipes in Mixes)
1 cup onion, chopped
1 teaspoon Seasoned Salt (see recipe in Mixes)
1/2 teaspoon ground mustard
1/2 teaspoon garlic powder
1/4 teaspoon pepper
1/4 teaspoon rubbed sage
1/4 teaspoon ground celery seed

Kitchen Tools:
Medium bowl
Measuring cups and spoons
Loaf pan
Cutting board and your favorite chopping knife

Instructions:

1. Preheat oven to 350 degrees F (177 degrees C). Line loaf pan with foil and then spray with oil. Set aside.
2. In a medium bowl, combine all ingredients. Use your hands to mix well or use a mixer with dough hooks.
3. Pack lightly but evenly into the loaf pan and bake for 1 hour to 1 hour 15 minutes, until loaf is cooked in the center.
4. Serve plain or with Red Bell Pepper Sauce (see recipe in Sauces)

Pot Roast

Any dish we can fix and forget while we go to work is a sure winner. There's nothing like coming home to a house that smells like someone has been slaving over a hot stove all day. We spend a lot of time in the kitchen, and anything we can do to free us up to have fun is a bonus.

The simplicity of the ingredients makes this dish especially attractive to us, and is reminiscent of the delicious hardiness of farm food. It's a complete meal without fuss, and all the prep time is on the front end, which you control. If you like, put this together the night before, refrigerate in the crock pot, and turn it on in the morning before you leave for work. June

Serves: 4
Prep Time: 45 minutes
Cook Time: 8 to 10 hours

Ingredients:
3 lbs. round roast
5 carrots, cut in 2" pieces
3 stalks celery, cut in 2" pieces
2 medium potatoes, cut in 2" pieces
1 large sweet onion, halved and cut into 1" chunks
1/2 lb. parsnips, cut in 2" pieces

---

1 cup salt free Beef Broth (see recipe in Mixes)
1/4 cup Bette Hagman's Featherlight Flour Mix (see recipe in Mixes)
1/3 cup Onion Soup & Dip Mix (see recipe in Mixes)

Kitchen Tools:
Crock Pot
Vegetable peeler
Cutting board
Your favorite chef's knife

Instructions:

1. Oil crockpot and place roast in first.
2. Peel and cut vegetables as specified and place around meat.
3. Measure beef broth into a small bowl and stir in flour and onion soup mix until dissolved. Pour over meat and vegetables, and cover crockpot. Cook on low for 8 to 10 hours.
4. If liquid generated is too thin for your liking, pour the hot broth into a pan. Dissolve a bit of cornstarch in a small amount of cold water and pour into broth, heating over medium heat and stirring constantly until it reaches the desired consistency.

Seasoned Hamburgers

Kris and I have become so accustomed to cooking and fearlessly attempting any new dish, that it came as a surprise to me to discover that a lot of people we talked with, do not cook past opening a microwaveable package. When putting this cookbook together, we determined early on that we would make it as user-friendly as possible. For that reason, we have included a basic recipe for hamburgers that are juicy and tasty. As with all recipes, feel free to make adjustments and additions that suit your taste. June

Serves: 4
Prep Time: 20 minutes
Cook Time: 8 minutes

Ingredients:

1 lb. lean ground beef
1 egg
1/2 cup gluten free bread crumbs
1 sweet onion, chopped
3/4 teaspoon Seasoned Salt (see recipe in Mixes)
2 teaspoons non-salt seasoning such as Mrs. Dash

Kitchen Tools:

Medium bowl
Measuring cups and spoons
Large griddle or skillet
Your hands for mixing

Instructions:

1. Combine all ingredients in a medium bowl and mix well. Your hands work best for this task.
2. Divide mixture into four equal parts and form each into a large, thin paddy. Place on a heated, dry griddle or skillet. There's no need to use additional oil, as the ground beef will supply that. Paddy will shrink a bit and plump up as it cooks.
3. Cook 4 minutes on each side for medium well-done hamburgers. Serve on Burger Buns (see recipe in Breads) or without bread, topped with Red Bell Pepper Sauce (see recipe in Sauces).

CHICKEN

Chickens are amazing creatures with individual personalities and a social hierarchy. My sister-in-law has six chickens at her quiet country home in Minnesota, which she has raised since they were barely out of the egg. They know her voice and respond to their names when called, especially at feeding time.

When her outside cat had kittens in the wintertime, the warm hen house and the egg nests became a new home for Mama Kitty and her babies. To everyone's amazement, Mama Kitty secured a surrogate mother when she went out mousing. Alpha Hen could be seen with the kittens under her wings in the nest, keeping them warm and safe. As they grew older, Alpha Hen would try to coax the kittens back in the hen house every evening.

Chickens display wonderful nurturing qualities, which is often reflected in the comfort and joy chicken dishes can provide. Chicken is considered a comfort food, especially if you are not feeling well.

The dishes in this section have been developed with taste, variety and texture in mind. Some are old favorites: Chicken Pot Pie, Chicken Rice Bake, and Chicken Nuggets. You'll find Chicken Crepes With Mixed Vegetables & Parsley, and Chicken Piccata With Artichokes Hearts to be elegant dishes to serve your guests. These recipes will enable you to enjoy chicken like you've never had it before.

Chicken Crepes With Mixed Vegetables & Parsley

This recipe was born out of a desire for a light, elegant dish with gentle flavors. In my younger years, I was a server in a high-end restaurant in Brattleboro, Vermont that served crepes when they were all the rage. I still occasionally see crepes on restaurant menus, but I personally believe they are a highly underrated food.

While it might seem like there are a lot of steps to this dish, don't be intimidated by the different components. Each part is manageable, and the end result is a dish for which you would gladly pay big money in an upscale restaurant. June

Serves: 6

Prep and Cook Time: 2 hours (but so worth it!)

Ingredients:

2 tablespoons oil

1 large onion, diced

4 chicken breasts, cut into 1" pieces

1 1/2 teaspoons non-salt seasoning such as Mrs. Dash

1 teaspoon Seasoned Salt (see recipe in Mixes)

---

2 cups frozen, mixed vegetables

2 to 3 tablespoons water

1/2 teaspoon Mrs. Dash or other non-salt spice

---

1 serving Crepe Cream Sauce (see recipe in Sauces)

1/2 cup chopped fresh parsley

Incredible Crepes (see recipe in Breads)

Kitchen Tools:

Cutting board and sharp knife

Medium sized skillet

1 1/2-quart saucepan

Measuring cups and spoons

Instructions:

1. In medium skillet, heat oil for a minute over medium heat. Add onion, chicken, salt-free spice, and seasoned salt, and continue cooking, stirring often until onions are soft and chicken is cooked through.
2. When chicken is cooked, turn up heat a bit, stirring often to keep chicken from burning, and reduce the liquid in the pan through evaporation. This process will intensify the flavors.
3. Meanwhile, in a saucepan, cook the mixed vegetables in 2 to 3 tablespoons water with the non-salt seasoning. Cover tightly and cook over medium heat until vegetables are just tender but not mushy, about 5 to 7 minutes. Stir often and watch so they don't burn.
4. Prepare the crepe sauce and mix into the chicken mixture, along with the chopped parsley and cooked vegetables. Set aside and keep warm.
5. Make the crepes one by one, remove them to a plate, and cover with a cloth to keep warm and pliable.
6. To construct crepes, place one crepe on a plate. Spoon approximately 3 tablespoons of the chicken mixture onto the lower half of the crepe. Fold the bottom 1/3 of the crepe up, fold right side and left side in, and roll the crepe up from the bottom, with the seam side down. If desired, spoon a little sauce over the top. Serve warm.

Tip: If possible, have two 6" nonstick skillets going at the same time to make the crepes. It will cut your crepe cooking time in half. Better yet, get older kids involved. At 13 years old, my grandson loves making crepes, especially the part about flipping the crepe without using a spatula. Move over, Emeril!

Tip: Fill leftover crepes with ice cream, served with a bit of chocolate agave (if tolerated) over the top, or fill with fresh fruit topped with sweetened, chilled coconut cream.

Chicken Croquettes

We had three cups of cooked chicken in the freezer, nothing planned for dinner, and it was chicken night on our rotation plan. We had made vegetable croquettes but never ventured into a meat-based croquette. We consulted The Flavor Bible by Karen Page and Andrew Dornenburg, published by Little, Brown and Company, copyright 2008 and combined our favorite herbs for this easy to make dish. If you have a large electric skillet that will accommodate all 14 croquettes, you will cut the cooking time in half. Kris

Makes: 14 croquettes
Prep Time: 35 minutes
Cook Time: 20 to 30 minutes

Ingredients:

2 tablespoons grapeseed oil
2 cups finely chopped onion

---

2 garlic cloves, minced

---

3 cups cooked chicken*

---

2 eggs, lightly beaten

---

1 cup dry bread crumbs
1/4 cup Daiya Mozzarella Style Shreds cheese
1/4 cup fresh chopped parsley
2 teaspoons Seasoned Salt (see recipe in Mixes)
1 teaspoon Garlic & Herb Mrs. Dash Chicken seasoning
1 teaspoon Table Blend Mrs. Dash
1/2 teaspoon ground black pepper
1/4 teaspoon marjoram
1/4 teaspoon savory
1/4 teaspoon sage

---

4 additional tablespoons grapeseed oil for griddle

Kitchen Tools:

Food Processor or chopper

Measuring cups and spoons

Garlic press

Small skillet

Large griddle

Stand mixer with dough hooks

Instructions:

1. Heat oil in skillet and add the chopped onion. Cook over medium heat, stirring often, until onions are translucent. Add the garlic and cook for an additional minute. Transfer to mixer bowl.
2. Using a food processor or food chopper, process chicken until finely chopped. Add to mixer bowl.
3. Break eggs into a small bowl and beat lightly. Add to mixer bowl.
4. Add the bread crumbs, Daiya cheese, parsley, seasoned salt, Mrs. Dash, pepper, marjoram, savory, and sage. Using dough hooks, mix on high for 2 minutes to incorporate all flavors and encourage a cohesive texture.
5. Mixture will be sticky but you have some choices. You can coat your hands with oil and, using a light hand, form into patties less than 1/2" thick and about 3" to 4" across. Another option is to oil two pieces of plastic wrap and form the patties between the plastic.
6. Heat 2 tablespoons of grapeseed oil in griddle over medium heat and, when hot, reduce heat to medium low. Fry patties on the hot griddle for 5 minutes on each side. Keep warm in the oven while you repeat the process until all croquettes are cooked.

*If you don't have cooked chicken on hand, use boneless chicken breasts, diced and stir-fried until cooked through.

Chicken Nuggets

One of the foods my grandson missed the most, when we discovered he was gluten intolerant, was chicken nuggets. Kris had already been on a gluten-free diet for months, and was also struggling with the additional dietary restrictions her allergies dictated, so when we discovered we could once again have chicken nuggets, there were some huge smiles around the table.

We began with a recipe from the glutenfreeclub.com, a great resource that offers an immense recipe data base, and features experts disseminating information in an easy-to-understand way. We adjusted quantities and ingredients to suit our allergies and taste. The end product is tasty chicken morsels with a crunchy outer coating. June

Serves: 4

Prep Time: 45 minutes

Cook Time: 35 minutes

Ingredients:

2 lbs. chicken breasts, cut into strips 3/4" wide and 1" long

---

High-heat oil for deep frying (canola, rice bran, safflower, sunflower)

Batter Ingredients:

1 large egg
1/2 cup brown rice flour
1/4 cup rice milk or hemp milk
1/4 cup tapioca flour
1 teaspoon Seasoned Salt (see recipe in Mixes)
1/2 teaspoon black pepper

Outer Coating Ingredients:

2 cups finely crushed potato, vegetable crisps*, tortilla chips, or crunchy cereal
2 tablespoons dried parsley
2 tablespoons plus 1 teaspoon Baking Powder (see recipe in Mixes)
1 tablespoon dried basil
2 teaspoons garlic powder
1 1/2 teaspoons Seasoned Salt
1 teaspoon savory
1 teaspoon dried oregano
1 teaspoon ground rosemary

* Snyder's Natural Garden Veggie Crisps work well, but if using, reduce seasoned salt to 1 teaspoon.

Kitchen Tools:

Handheld mixer or whisk

Small bowls

Resealable gallon plastic bag

Measuring cups and spoons

Pan for deep-frying (a wok works well)

Slotted spoon, perforated ladle or skimmer

Instructions:

1. In a small bowl, combine the batter ingredients, and beat with handheld mixer or whisk until well mixed. Set aside.
2. In a resealable plastic bag, combine the outer coating ingredients and shake to mix.
3. Cut chicken into strips, blot dry with a paper towel, and dip in the batter. Transfer chicken to the outer coating mix in the plastic bag, seal bag, and shake to coat.
4. Heat oil in a heavy pan over medium heat. To test the temperature, place a wooden chopstick upright in the center of the oil, and if oil bubbles up, you're ready to fry.
5. Fry chicken in batches until nuggets are golden brown, being careful not to crowd them in the pan. To test for doneness, remove a piece and cut it open. If there's any pink, return to the pan and continue to fry for at least another minute. Drain fried chicken on paper towels and keep warm in the oven until all nuggets have been cooked.
6. Serve warm. Leftovers are also great cold.

Chicken Piccata With Artichoke Hearts

This recipe was inspired by an unintentional stay at The Inn at Water's Edge in Ludlow, Vermont, during Hurricane Irene in August 2011. A friend and I were on vacation, and our immediate introduction to Ludlow was the necessity to drive through rising flood waters, as creeks and streams overran their banks. Water poured off the mountains, turning tarred and unpaved streets into water chutes. We were rescued by locals in a pickup, who took us to a hotel at an intersection of rushing water due to a dam break. We waded through moving water up to our knees, carrying our luggage, only to be told once we were safe on the hotel porch, that the hotel was under mandatory evacuation. Kind strangers transported us to an inn on higher ground across the bridge.

The Inn at Water's Edge is an elegant, New England inn, run by an engaging husband and wife who are funnier than a professional comedy team. Although they had not planned on guests for the weekend, Tina whipped together a fabulous meal for 15, featuring Chicken Piccata With Artichoke Hearts. This recipe was my best attempt to reconstruct her dish from taste bud memory. June

Serves: 4

Prep Time: 25 minutes

Cook Time: 15 minutes

Ingredients:

1 1/2 lbs. boneless chicken breasts, halved lengthwise or chicken tenderloins

---

2 tablespoons buttery spread

1 tablespoon grapeseed oil

Salt and pepper

1/4 cup plus 2 tablespoons fresh lemon juice

1/2 can artichoke hearts, drained

---

3 tablespoons minced fresh parsley

Kitchen Tools:

Cutting board

Sharp knife

Large skillet

Measuring spoons

Meat tenderizing mallet with a flat side

Instructions:

1. Slice chicken breasts lengthwise to give you pieces less than 1/2" thick. If necessary, place chicken slices or chicken tenderloins between plastic wrap, and gently pound to thin out to 1/4" thick.
2. Melt buttery spread and grapeseed oil in a large skillet over medium high heat. Sauté the chicken pieces, seasoned with salt and pepper, for 2 to 4 minutes on each side, or until they are just cooked through. Transfer to a plate.
3. Pour fresh lemon juice in the skillet, and stir to incorporate chicken drippings. Stir and heat, adding the chicken pieces, turning to coat.
4. Cut artichoke hearts in half lengthwise, add to skillet, and heat. Serve hot with fresh parsley sprinkled on top.

Chicken Quinoa With Asparagus

Quinoa is a wonderful grain that will take on the flavor of anything you combine with it, and makes the perfect base for a chicken dish. This recipe was the result of a desire to incorporate more of the perfect protein of quinoa into our diet, and to use up some of the chicken we had in the freezer. The addition of asparagus for color and nutrition, proved to be a good choice. Best of all, it's a quick, easy meal for busy people. Kris

Serves: 4
Prep Time: 15 minutes
Cook Time: 45 minutes

Ingredients:

1 tablespoon olive oil
1 large onion, chopped
1 lb. boneless chicken, cut into 1" pieces

---

1 cup quinoa, washed
1 1/4 cups salt free Chicken Broth (see recipe in Mixes)
1 1/4 teaspoons salt
2 garlic cloves, minced

---

1 tablespoon oil
1 lb. asparagus, washed and cut into 1" pieces

1/4 to 1/2 cup fresh basil leaves, slivered

Kitchen Tools:

Large skillet
Measuring cups and spoons
Splatter screen
Medium skillet
Cutting board and your favorite chopping knife

Instructions:

1. Heat oil in large skillet and add onion and chicken. Sauté over medium high heat, for about 7 minutes, stirring often, until onions are translucent and chicken is cooked through.
2. Meanwhile, measure quinoa into a bowl and fill with cold water. Swish quinoa around with your hand to remove the bitter coating. Place a splatter screen securely over the top of the bowl and drain the water. Repeat this process two more times. Add cleaned quinoa to the skillet along with the chicken broth, salt, and garlic.
3. Heat on high until mixture boils, and then reduce heat to low, cover tightly, and let simmer for 15 to 20 minutes. Check the quinoa often in the last 10 minutes to ensure it doesn't burn.
4. Meanwhile, heat oil in a medium skillet and add asparagus. Salt lightly and with heat on medium, stir-fry for 4 minutes, stirring often. Cover skillet and continue to cook for 2 minutes, until asparagus is barely tender. Set aside.
5. When quinoa is done, stir to separate and "fluff" the quinoa. Add the quinoa, asparagus and fresh basil to the chicken. Stir to combine and serve hot.

Variations:

Parsley Option: In the final stage, replace the fresh basil with 1/2 cup fresh parsley, washed and chopped.

Broccoli Option: Substitute fresh or frozen broccoli for the asparagus by adding 1/4 teaspoon dried basil to the chicken broth. Steam broccoli separately until done to your liking, and stir into quinoa in step 5. Eliminate the fresh basil leaves and add 1/2 cup fresh parsley.

G'ma's Chicken Pot Pie

I'm proud to admit I'm a great-grandmother. Life doesn't get any better than holding your great-grandbaby. With the arrival of little Emily, my granddaughter asked me what I wanted to be called and I drew a blank. With the number of grandparents, step-grandparents, and great-grandparents involved in this birth, the cool names like Nana, Mema, Grams, and Grandma were all taken, but I became known as G'ma, an affectionate name easy for a young tongue to say. That's a long explanation for how this recipe got its name.

I have always loved chicken pot pie, but had never tasted one that was homemade. I grew up on Swanson's Pot Pies, and after going gluten free, I missed the creamy gravy filling within the pie crust. My family graciously ate the many renditions until this recipe finally reached perfection. It's not a quick dish to make, but you could cut down on time by using frozen mixed vegetables in place of the fresh carrots, celery, and onions, with minimal sacrifice of flavor. However, the time spent making this comfort food is well worth the effort, and leftovers can be frozen! June

Serves: 6 to 8
Prep Time: 2 hours 30 minutes
Bake Time: 25 to 35 minutes

Ingredients for Filling:

2 lbs. boneless chicken breasts, cut into 1" pieces
5 cups salt free Chicken Broth (see recipe in Mixes)
1 large bay leaf

---

1 cup green beans, cut into 1/2" pieces
1 teaspoon ground thyme or savory

---

3 cups onion, chopped
2 cups carrots, peeled and cut into 3/8" slices
1 cup celery, cut into 3/8" slices

---

2 medium potatoes, cut into 1/2" cubes
2 garlic cloves, minced

---

1 3/4 cups rice milk

1/2 cup arrowroot starch

---

2 teaspoons Seasoned Salt (see recipe in Mixes)

1/4 teaspoon ground pepper

1/2 cup fresh parsley, minced

Ingredients for Crust:

2 1/4 cups brown rice flour

3/4 cup potato starch

1/4 cup plus 2 tablespoons arrowroot starch

1 1/2 teaspoons salt

1 1/2 teaspoons xanthan gum

---

1 cup plus 2 tablespoons Spectrum shortening

---

2 eggs, beaten

3 tablespoons fresh lemon juice

Kitchen Tools:

4 1/2-quart saucepan or larger

Measuring cups and spoons

Deep dish pie pan or individual baking dishes or a combination

Stand mixer

Medium bowl

Small bowl

Rolling pin

Plastic wrap

Instructions for Filling:

1. Oil baking dish(es) or pie pan and set aside. Preheat oven to 400 degrees F (204 degrees C) when the time is appropriate.
2. Place cut up chicken and chicken broth in saucepan and heat to boiling. Reduce heat to medium high and simmer for 10 minutes until chicken is tender. Remove chicken with a slotted spoon and set aside.
3. Put green beans and ground thyme or savory in chicken broth, cover, and boil for 5 minutes.
4. Add the onion, carrots, and celery. Cover and boil for 5 minutes.
5. Add the potatoes and garlic. Cover and cook about 5 minutes, until potatoes are tender but not mushy.
6. Stir arrowroot starch into rice milk until dissolved, and add to boiling vegetables. Stir constantly over medium heat until thickened. Remove and discard bay leaf.
7. Add the seasoned salt, pepper, and parsley, as well as the cooked chicken. Stir to combine. Set aside but keep warm while you make the pie crust.

Instructions for Crust:

8. Measure shortening and place in the freezer for a short time, or the refrigerator for a longer time, to chill well before using. Do not let the shortening freeze.
9. Wash and juice the lemon. Measure the juice and set aside.
10. Measure brown rice flour, potato starch, arrowroot starch, salt, and xanthan gum into the mixer bowl or food processor. Mix well.
11. Add the cold shortening to the flour mix, and pulse just until flour and shortening form beads or, better yet, use a pastry blender. Remove to a bowl if you've used a food processor.
12. In a small bowl, whisk together the egg and lemon juice. Add to the flour mix and stir just until mixture forms into a ball.
13. Spritz a bit of water on the counter. Tear off 1 piece of plastic wrap about 24" long. Place on counter and smooth it out. The water will hold it in place. Divide dough in two and cover one half to keep it moist. Form one half into a flattened ball and put in the middle of the wrap. **Note:** If your baking dish is square or rectangular in shape, form the dough into a square or rectangle before rolling. Smooth another piece of wrap over the flattened dough and using your rolling pin, roll outward from the center to thin out the dough. Dough should not be paper thin—no thinner than 1/8" and a little less than 1/4". Peel the top plastic wrap off the dough. If you are using individual baking dishes,

invert one of the dishes over the rolled out dough and press down to cut the dough just large enough to cover your baking dish. Continue this process until you have cut as many rounds as possible.

14. Cut the plastic wrap between the rounds with a scissor to make the dough easier to work with. Fill baking dishes with hot chicken mixture making sure to leave at least 1/2" to 3/4" at the top for expansion.
15. Peel the bottom plastic wrap up from the counter, being careful not to tear the pie crust. Supporting it with your other hand, gently turn it over and center the crust on top of the baking dish. Gently peel the plastic wrap from the crust, and smooth it at the edges and up against the inside wall of the dish. Crust will be simply sitting on top of the hot filling. Prick crust in several places to vent steam, and place baking dishes on a cookie sheet in case filling over tops.
16. Bake for 25 to 35 minutes until crust is slightly browned. Remove from oven and let rest for a few minutes before serving.

Note: If you're using frozen chicken and frozen broth, cut down on your prep time by thawing in advance. You can also prepare carrots, celery, and onions in advance when you have a free block of time.

Variations:

Mashed Potato Crust: If your time is at a premium, you can substitute mashed potatoes for the pie crust. Do not change the bake time.

Quick Garlic Chicken & Parsley

We were hungry for the combination of Gnocchi, chicken, and garlic. Because Gnocchi is not a quick dish to make, we needed a garlic chicken we could put in the oven and forget while the Gnocchi were being prepared. The ingredients for the chicken are uncomplicated and quick to put together. The results are pungent and go perfectly with Gnocchi (see recipe in Pasta). Kris

Serves: 4
Prep Time: 10 minutes
Bake Time: 40 minutes

Ingredients:
2 lbs. chicken cutlets
2/3 cup olive oil
6 garlic cloves, minced
1 1/4 teaspoons Seasoned Salt (see recipe in Mixes)

1/2 cup fresh parsley, chopped

Kitchen Tools:
Measuring cup and spoon
Garlic press
8" x 8" baking dish
Small bowl

Instructions:

1. Preheat oven to 350 degrees F (177 degrees C). Oil baking dish and arrange chicken cutlets in a single layer.
2. In a small bowl, stir together garlic, olive oil, and seasoned salt. Pour over chicken and bake uncovered for 40 minutes.
3. Remove from oven and sprinkle parsley over chicken. We love it served over Gnocchi, but you could make do with your favorite pasta or cooked rice.

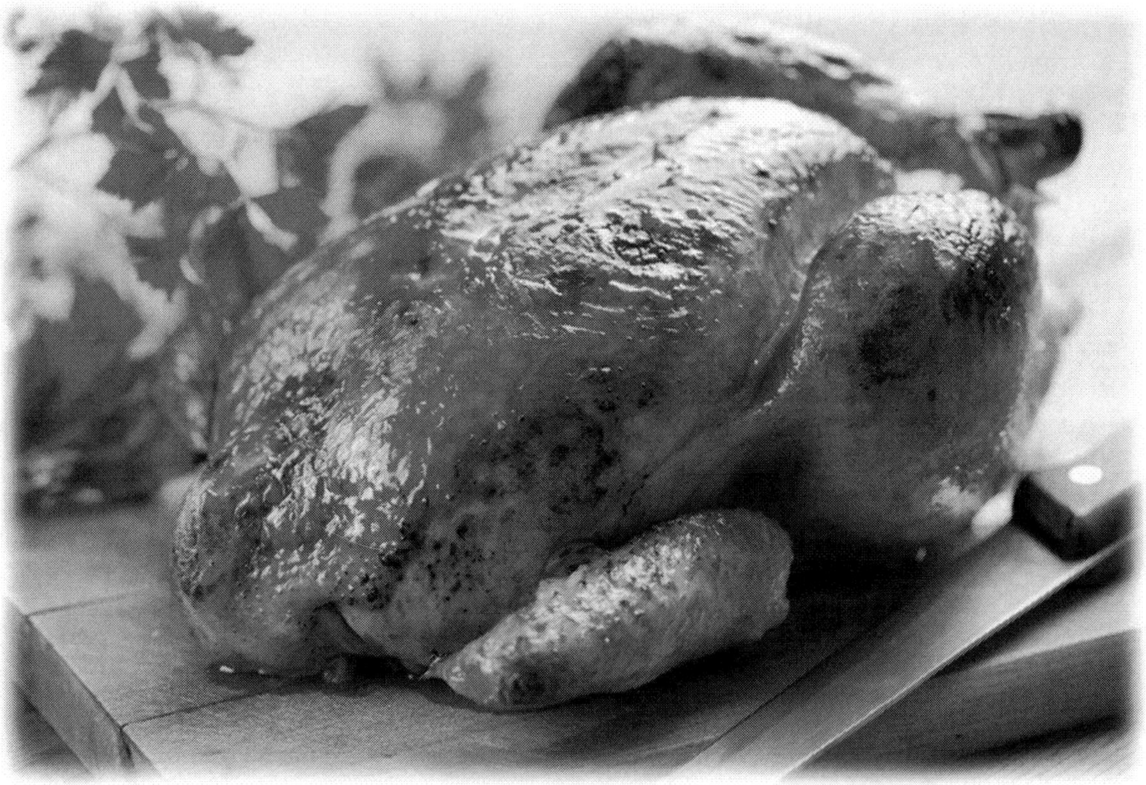

Lemon Mint Chicken & Potatoes

While dried mint is one of the herbs used in this dish, its effect is subtle in combination with the oregano, salt, and pepper. Lemon juice mixed with the chicken broth lends just the right amount of zest, and the addition of the chopped red bell pepper tops off this dish with beautiful color. Red skinned potatoes will give you the best results.

This dish was minimally reworked from a recipe in the Wheat-Free, Gluten-Free Cookbook for Kids and Busy Adults, Second Edition (2010), by Connie Sarros and offered here with her permission. We urge you to check out her excellent cookbook for recipes you may be able to adapt. Kris

Serves: 4
Prep Time: 30 minutes
Bake Time: 1 hour 30 minutes

Ingredients:

1 1/2 lbs. chicken cutlets

---

4 red-skinned potatoes

---

6 garlic cloves, quartered
1 lemon, juiced
1/2 cup salt free Chicken Broth (see recipe in Mixes)
1/4 cup olive oil
1/4 cup chopped red bell pepper
1 1/2 teaspoons dried oregano
1/2 teaspoon salt
1/2 teaspoon dried mint
1/4 teaspoon pepper

Kitchen Tools:

Measuring cups and spoons

8" x 11" baking dish

Small bowl

Citrus juicer

Instructions:

1. Preheat oven to 350 degrees F (177 degrees C). Oil baking dish and place chicken in dish.
2. Wash potatoes and slice in half lengthwise. Cut each half into no thicker than 1/2" slices, again lengthwise. Scatter around chicken.
3. Slice garlic cloves and put in small bowl. Add the remaining ingredients, stir well, and pour over chicken and potatoes.
4. Bake for 1 hour 30 minutes, stirring halfway through baking time. Flavor will be enhanced through occasional basting.
5. Serve with at least one vegetable side dish and enjoy!

Garlic Roasted Chicken

Sometimes we want the convenience of prepping for a meal when we have a block of time, and this dish is perfect for that. The marinade time can be flexible—up to 24 hours—and the end product is baked for only 45 minutes. The garlic is pronounced, but blends in well with the slight tartness of the lemon juice and the chicken broth. Feel free to reduce the lemon or cut it out altogether for a different taste. Either way, the baked juices can be served au jus or over your favorite pasta or rice. Kris

Serves: 4
Prep Time: 30 minutes
Marinating Time: 4 to 24 hours
Bake Time: 45 minutes

Ingredients:
2 lbs. chicken cutlets

Marinade Ingredients:
1/2 cup garlic cloves (approximately 1 1/2 bulbs)
2 cups salt free Chicken Broth (see recipe in Mixes)
2 tablespoons olive oil
1 tablespoon Seasoned Salt (see recipe in Mixes)
1/2 teaspoon black pepper

---

1 lemon, cut into wedges
2 bay leaves

Kitchen Tools:
Measuring cups and spoons
Large sealable plastic bag or glass bowl
8" x 11" baking dish
Small saucepan

Instructions:

1. Put garlic, chicken broth, olive oil, seasoned salt, and pepper in a blender. Blend on high for 2 minutes. Pour into plastic bag or bowl.
2. Wash lemon and cut the long way into 8 wedges. Remove seeds and squeeze the lemon wedges into the broth mixture. Toss in the lemon and add the bay leaves.
3. Add chicken to the marinade and seal plastic bag or cover bowl. Refrigerate overnight or up to 24 hours.
4. Preheat oven to 375 degrees F (191 degrees C).
5. Remove chicken from marinade and place in baking dish. Discard the lemon wedges and bay leaves, and pour the marinade into a saucepan. Heat to a rolling boil to kill any bacteria, and continue to boil to reduce the liquid by 1/2, thereby intensifying the flavors. Pour redux over chicken and bake for 45 minutes, basting often with the marinade and juices.

Note: If using thicker pieces of chicken such as legs or breasts, adjust baking time accordingly.

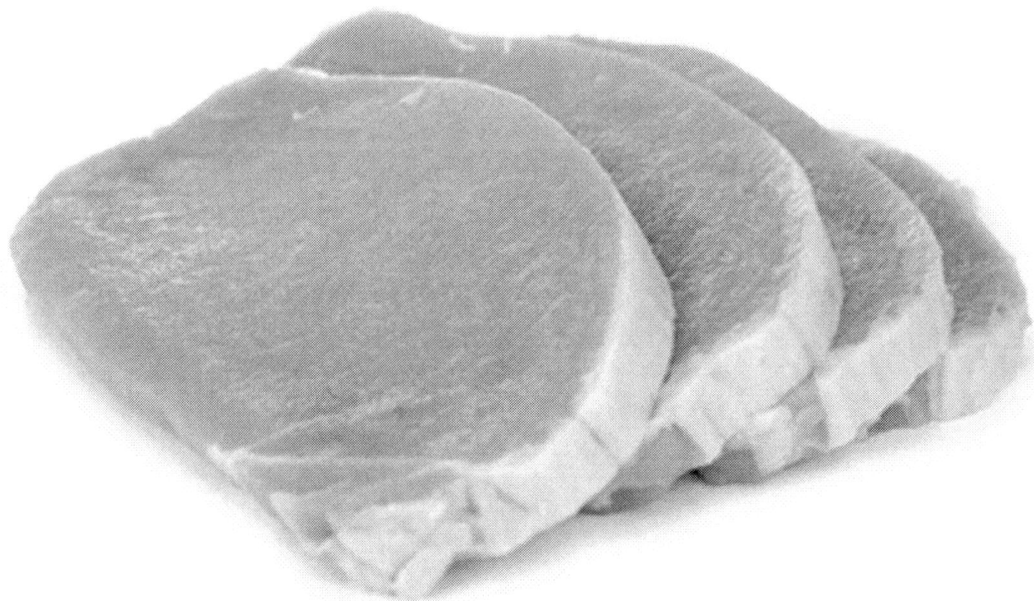

Pork

Growing up on a self-sustained dairy farm in Minnesota, gave me life experiences that formed my taste buds and expectations for the quality of my food, for the rest of my life. Our pigs were fed grain we grew, and food scraps from our table. Their water was pure, deep well water without chemicals, and the difference in the taste of the meat was amazing.

Using only the freshest beef and pork, my parents were master sausage makers. Bacon, hams, and sausages were carefully smoked in our own smokehouse, and hung to cure. It was not until I left home and had to purchase grocery store meat, that I realized how blessed I had been.

If you are able to purchase organic meats, do so and you'll be able to tell the difference.

Italian Herbed Pork Chops

This recipe is an adaptation of a recipe found on www.myspicesage.com and was designed for flank steak. We discovered the website in a search for ground celery seed, which we couldn't find in any local grocery store. They offer an amazing assortment of high-quality spices and herbs, and a gluten-free section. Herbs and spices are thoroughly described, including other common names, the taste or aroma category, and possible substitutions.

The multitude of dried herbs in this recipe gives the pork a wonderful, rich flavor. It requires marinating for at least an hour, but will be much better if marinated for 6 hours. Lean, thick, boneless pork chops are sliced against the grain, on a bias, to give you wider slices. This dish is pan-fried which allows the flavors to continue to cook into the meat for a tender, flavorful dish. Kris

Serves: 4
Prep Time: 15 minutes
Marinating Time: 1 to 8 hours
Cook Time: 15 to 20 minutes

Ingredients:

1 1/2 to 2 lbs. lean, boneless pork chops, thinly sliced (see note below on how to slice)

---

1 lemon, juiced
3 tablespoons olive oil
2 teaspoons garlic powder
1 1/4 teaspoons Seasoned Salt (see recipe in Mixes)
1/2 teaspoon ground rosemary
1/2 teaspoon ground marjoram
1/2 teaspoon oregano
1/2 teaspoon paprika
1/2 teaspoon black pepper
1/2 teaspoon ground savory

---

3 tablespoons oil
1 large onion, quartered and sliced

Kitchen Tools:

Large bowl

Whisk

Measuring spoon

Citrus juicer

Large skillet

Instructions:

1. For the greatest ease in slicing, wrap chops in plastic wrap and place in your freezer for 45 minutes. Remove from the freezer, discard the plastic wrap, and cut off any fat. Cut the chops in thin slices by cutting against the grain and on the bias. If you're unsure what that means, lay the chops out on a cutting board and look at the way the grain goes—and position the meat so the grain runs horizontally to you. Cutting on the bias is achieved by placing your knife at a 45-degree angle and slicing across the grain. This will give you wider slices than if your knife was straight up and down, increasing the area to be marinated, and aiding in creating more tenderness.
2. In a medium bowl large enough to marinate all the meat, whisk together the lemon juice, olive oil, garlic powder, seasoned salt, rosemary, marjoram, oregano, paprika, pepper, and savory. Mix well and add the sliced pork. Stir to ensure all meat is coated, cover bowl, and refrigerate for up to 8 hours.
3. Heat 3 tablespoons oil in a large skillet over medium high heat and add onion. Stir-fry briefly.
4. Pour meat and marinade into skillet and cover. Reduce heat if necessary so it doesn't burn, and continue to cook, stirring occasionally for 15 to 20 minutes, until onions are browned and liquid is reduced. Serve hot.

Marinated Pork Stir-Fry

The many various sources on the internet generally agree that stir-fry originated in China, but exact origins or reasons are a bit vague. One account declares stir-fry was invented out of a need for fast cooking, because fuel was always in short supply. For whatever reason, stir-fry is a great way to add a lot of vegetables into your meal. The pork is marinated and, when cooked, retains the flavor of the marinade. This is especially good served over jasmine rice. Kris

Serves: 6
Prep Time: 30 minutes
Marinating Time: 3 to 12 hours
Cook Time: 20 minutes

Ingredients:

3 pork chops, thinly sliced in 1" pieces, fat removed
Juice of 1 lemon
1/3 cup salt free Beef Broth (see recipe in Mixes)
1 tablespoon Herbes De Provence
1 tablespoon non-salt seasoning such as Mrs. Dash
1 teaspoon Seasoned Salt (see recipe in Mixes)
4 garlic cloves, minced

---

1 tablespoon Stir Fry Tea Oil or other high-heat oil

---

2 tablespoons Stir Fry Tea Oil or other high-heat oil
3 carrots, thinly sliced diagonally
3 stalks celery, thinly sliced diagonally

---

1 bunch scallions, sliced
1 red, yellow or orange pepper, seeded and cut in strips
1 medium zucchini, sliced
1/2 teaspoon Seasoned Salt

---

1 can sliced water chestnuts, drained

---

2 tablespoons cornstarch
1 cup salt free Beef Broth

Kitchen Tools:

Citrus juicer

Medium bowl

Measuring cups and spoons

Wok or large nonstick pan

Instructions:

1. In a medium bowl, mix together the pork, lemon juice, beef broth, Herbes De Provence, non-salt seasoning, seasoned salt, and garlic. Stir to combine, cover, and refrigerate for several hours or overnight if possible.
2. Prepare all vegetables and set aside as grouped.
3. Heat 1 tablespoon of oil in the wok over medium to high heat, and carefully add pork with any remaining marinade. Stir-fry about 10 minutes until pork is tender and most of the liquid has evaporated. Pour meat into a bowl and set aside.
4. Heat 2 tablespoons oil in the wok and add the carrots and celery. Stir-fry, stirring constantly for 3 minutes.
5. Add the scallions, pepper, zucchini, and seasoned salt. Continue to stir-fry for another 2 minutes.
6. Add the water chestnuts and fry for 1 minute until vegetables are just tender.
7. Dissolve cornstarch in cold beef broth, and pour into the center of the wok, stirring constantly until thickened. Add pork that has been set aside and stir to combine. Serve over rice.

Pork Curry

Curry has a rich history, with a recipe for curry appearing on cuneiform text, discovered by the Sumerians, and dated around 1700 BC in Babylon in Mesopotamia. During the reign of Richard II in England, the first real English cookery book was written in 1390 with a reference to curry. It wasn't until 1780 that the first commercial curry powder was introduced. (Curry, Spice & All Things Nice) Today, you'll find as many recipes for curry as there are families who make it.

I readily admit that I didn't like curry, or thought I didn't, until Kris whipped up this meal one evening. When I walked through the door, the aroma was wonderful and made my mouth water. Much to my delight, I loved the mild taste and spices in this dish, which works equally well with chicken. It's best served over brown rice but we've also used a base of pasta or spaghetti squash. June

Serves: 4
Prep Time: 20 minutes
Cook Time: 25 minutes

Ingredients:

2 tablespoons oil

---

1 lb. pork loin or pork chops, thinly sliced and fat removed
2 large white onions, chopped
1 teaspoon salt
1/8 teaspoon pepper

---

1 tablespoon curry powder
1 teaspoon cumin
1/2 teaspoon coriander
1/2 teaspoon turmeric
1/4 teaspoon cinnamon
2 garlic cloves, minced

---

1 cup salt free Beef Broth (see recipe in Mixes)
1/2 cup coconut milk
2 tablespoons Bette Hagman's Modified GF Flour Mix (see recipe in Mixes)
10 drops SweetLeaf Valencia Orange liquid stevia

Kitchen Tools:

Skillet

Measuring cups and spoons

Cutting board

Sharp knife

Instructions:

1. Heat oil in the skillet and add the pork, onions, salt, and pepper. Fry over medium heat just until pork is no longer pink, and onions are translucent. Don't overfry.
2. Add the curry powder, cumin, coriander, turmeric, cinnamon, and garlic. Stir and cook for 1 minute longer.
3. Combine the beef broth, coconut milk, flour, and liquid stevia, stirring to dissolve the flour. Pour liquid into the skillet, scraping up the browned bits. Bring to a boil, reduce heat, cover, and gently simmer for 15 minutes, stirring often.
4. Serve over brown rice.

Variations:

Chicken Curry: Substitute chicken breasts, cut into 1" cubes, and substitute chicken broth for the beef broth.

Curry with Carrots and Potatoes: Add 1 cup cooked carrots and 1 cup cubed, cooked potatoes to the finished dish.

Works Cited

Curry, Spice & All Things Nice: The History of Curry by Peter & Colleen Grove. http://www.menumagazine.co.uk/book/curryhistory.html. Retrieved January 27, 2013.

Sunflower Crusted Pork Chops

These pork chops go together in 20 minutes or less, and then spend the next hour and a half blissfully baking, not needing any attention, while you go about your duties. When they emerge from the oven, they have a wonderful crust and a tender, delicious center you can almost cut with your fork.

We've used sunflower seeds here, but if you can tolerate pistachios, they also make a great coating. Pistachios are of the same family as mango and cashews, but all research we have seen agrees that it is possible to be allergic to cashews but not pistachios, or vice versa. Some people are allergic to all tree nuts as well as peanuts, so you must use your own best judgment in all things. Kris

Serves: 3
Prep Time: 20 minutes
Bake Time: 1 hour 30 minutes

Ingredients:

3 pork chops, 3/4" to 1" thick

1/2 cup roasted sunflower seeds, finely ground
1/2 cup ground gluten free puffed rice cereal, crackers or tortilla chips
1/2 teaspoon Seasoned Salt (see recipe in Mixes)
1/2 teaspoon ground mustard

---

1 egg
1 1/2 teaspoons water
1 1/2 teaspoons Italian Herb Mix (see recipe in Mixes)
1/2 teaspoon Seasoned Salt
1/2 teaspoon garlic powder
1/4 teaspoon ground pepper

Kitchen Tools:

8" x 11" baking dish

Food processor

Measuring cups and spoons

Shallow bowl

Small bowl

Whisk

Instructions:

1. Preheat oven to 350 degrees F (177 degrees C). Oil baking dish and set aside.
2. Using a food processor, grind sunflower seeds to a fine consistency. Pour into a shallow bowl. Repeat the process with the puffed rice cereal and add to the bowl. Add seasoned salt, ground mustard, and stir to combine.
3. In a small bowl, whisk together the egg, water, Italian herb mix, seasoned salt, garlic powder, and pepper.
4. Dip pork chops in egg mixture and then press into the coating mix, covering both sides and edges of the pork chops. Place in baking dish and bake for 1 hour 30 minutes, until chops are cooked through and tender. There is no need to turn the chops during baking.

Variations:

Pistachio Crusted Pork Chops: If tolerated, substitute 1/2 cup pistachio nuts for the sunflower seeds, and follow remaining directions.

One Pot Pork

One pot meals are always a plus for busy people. Kris doesn't really like pork, so it's a challenge to camouflage the taste and still make it pleasing to the rest of the family. We have used simple, minimal ingredients to achieve an easy-to make, quick dish with texture, taste, and eye appeal. This dish passed not only the Kris test but also the kid test. We hope it brings a smile to your taste buds. June

Serves: 4
Prep Time: 40 minutes
Cook Time: 30 minutes

Ingredients:

1 lb. lean pork tenderloin or pork chops, cut into bite-sized pieces
1 1/2 cups salt free Chicken Broth (see recipe in Mixes)
1 cup uncooked long grain brown rice
1 tablespoon non-salt seasoning such as Mrs. Dash
1 tablespoon Herbs de Provence or Italian Herb Mix (see recipe in Mixes)
2 1/2 teaspoons Seasoned Salt (see recipe in Mixes)
1/4 teaspoon pepper

---

3 cups carrots, diced
3 stalks celery, diced
3 garlic cloves, minced

Kitchen Tools:

Large skillet
Bowl
Measuring cups and spoons
Cutting board
Your favorite chef's knife

Instructions:

1. Cut pork into bite-sized pieces and add to cold skillet. Add the chicken broth.
2. Measure brown rice into a bowl, fill with water, swish around, and drain well. Wash rice in this way two more times, draining well on the last wash. Add rice to the skillet.
3. Stir in the non-salt seasoning, Herbs de Provence, seasoned salt, and pepper. Bring to a boil and reduce heat to simmer. Cover and cook 20 minutes, stirring often.
4. Stir in carrots, celery, and garlic. Simmer for another 10 to 15 minutes until vegetables are soft and rice absorbs most of the liquid. Serve hot.

Variations:

White Rice Option: The seasonings and method of cooking are geared toward brown rice. If you use white rice, make sure it's long grain rice. Reduce Herbs de Provence to 1 teaspoon and add 1 teaspoon Chicken Grilling Blends by Mrs. Dash. Reduce cook time in step 3 to 15 minutes.

Herbed Pork Tenderloin

The seasoning on this meat is aromatic and wonderfully flavorful. This method of roasting is fast and, if not over roasted, the meat will be moist. The last 20 minutes of resting time allow the juices to settle in the meat for maximum moistness. Kris

Serves: 4
Prep Time: 10 minutes
Roasting Time: 1 hour
Rest Time: 20 minutes

Ingredients:

1/2 cup water

---

2 lbs. boneless pork loin, with fat on

---

1 tablespoon olive oil
1 1/2 teaspoons Seasoned Salt (see recipe in Mixes)
1 teaspoon garlic powder
1/2 teaspoon dried savory
1/2 teaspoon dried basil
1/2 teaspoon dried rosemary
1/2 teaspoon ground mustard

Kitchen Tools:

Baking pan
Small Bowl

Instructions:

1. Preheat oven to 475 degrees F (246 degrees C). Oil baking pan and add 1/2 cup water.
2. In a small bowl, stir together the olive oil, seasoned salt, garlic powder, savory, basil, rosemary, and ground mustard. Massage the mixture into the pork, covering all areas.
3. Place meat in baking pan and roast for 30 minutes. Reduce the heat to 425 degrees F (220 degrees C) and roast for an additional 30 minutes. If the juices in the bottom of the pan evaporate, add a bit of hot water or broth.
4. Remove pan from oven and let sit for 20 minutes before carving. It will continue to cook during that time. Temperature at the center of the meat must be at least 155 to be safe. Do not over roast, as the meat will dry out along with its flavor.

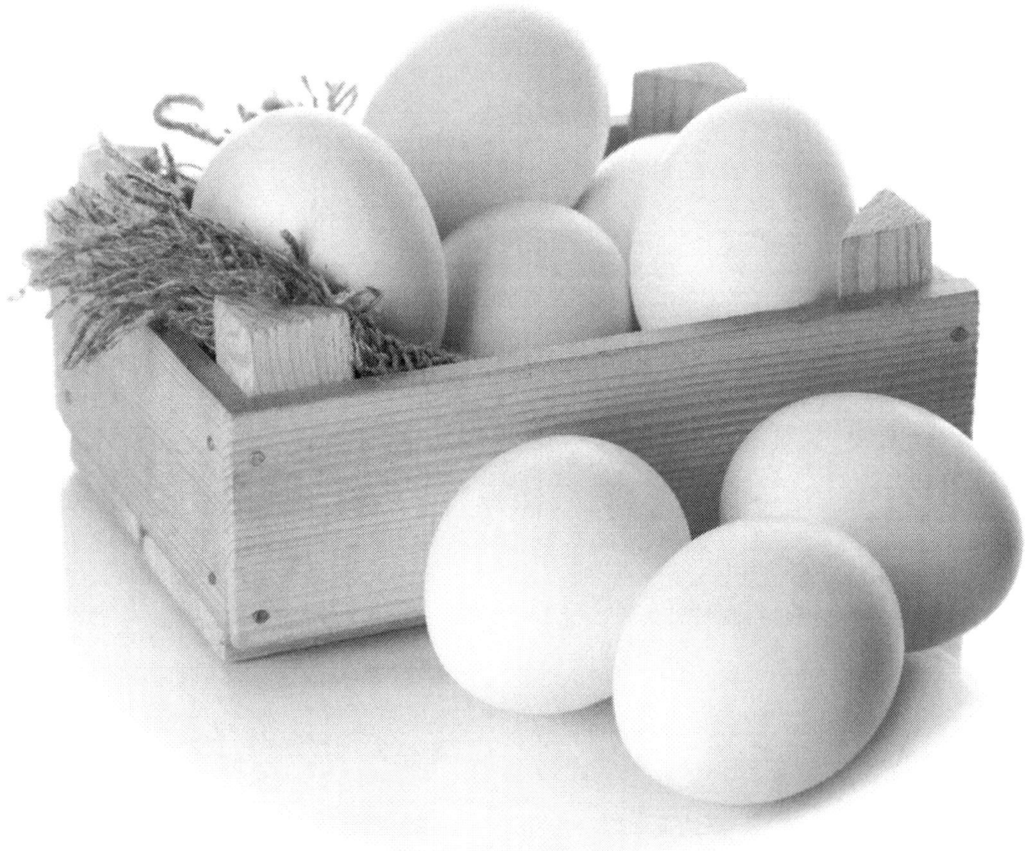

Eggs

Eggs are probably the most versatile food we have available to us. In their whole form, they can be a breakfast or a main course. They can be baked, fried, poached, microwaved, and combined with countless ingredients, giving us everything from down home simple food to exotic dishes with foreign spices. There are entire cookbooks dedicated to the egg and its incredible diversity.

With all the potential of the humble egg, you will only find five recipes in this section, but they are family favorites designed to give you fresh ideas for a meal. You can change the overall taste of any of these recipes by adding your favorite fresh herbs. Be creative, experiment, and write in the cookbook what works for you. Rediscover the joy of eggs.

Ham & Cheese Strata

Strata is typically an American dish of multiple layers (thus the name strata) of bread, eggs, meats, and/or vegetables. There's always a resting period of at least an hour and up to overnight, to allow bread and flavors to mingle before baking, which makes it the perfect breakfast or brunch dish. Ingredients can be as exotic or as simple as you like, so the possibilities of variety with the combination of ingredients and herbs is mind-boggling.

This dish is meant to be made in advance, so take advantage of the timing for a delicious main dish dinner or easy breakfast. June

Serves: 4
Prep Time: 30 minutes
Rest Time: 1 to 8 hours
Bake Time: 45 to 50 minutes

Ingredients:

6 to 8 slices gluten-free bread, sliced thin

---

1 cup ham, diced
1/4 cup scallions, sliced
1/4 cup red or orange bell peppers, diced
1/4 cup green peppers, diced
1/2 cup Daiya Cheddar Jack Cheese
1/2 cup Daiya Cheddar Style Shreds cheese

---

6 eggs
1 cup rice milk
1/2 cup Egg Beaters or other 0 fat egg product
1 teaspoon ground mustard
1 teaspoon non-salt seasoning
1 teaspoon Herbamare or Seasoned Salt (see recipe in Mixes)
1/4 teaspoon black pepper

Kitchen Tools:

9" x 13" baking dish

Measuring cups and spoons

Medium bowl

Whisk or handheld mixer

Instructions:

1. Oil baking dish and place bread in a single layer in the bottom.
2. Evenly sprinkle the ham, scallions, bell peppers, green peppers, and Daiya cheeses over the bread.
3. In a medium bowl, whisk together the eggs, rice milk, Egg Beaters, ground mustard, non-salt seasoning, Herbamare, and pepper. Pour over the bread and refrigerate for at least 1 hour and up to 8 hours.
4. Preheat oven to 350 degrees F (177 degrees C) when the time is right.
5. Bake for 45 to 50 minutes. Allow to rest for a few minutes before serving.

Bacon Onion Quiche

This quiche makes a wonderful dinner, served with a salad or freshly made rolls. Leftovers heat well in the microwave and are perfect for breakfast. If you are using turkey bacon, as suggested, there's no need to cook it first. If you use pork bacon, you will need to chop and panfry it just until cooked through, so allow some extra time. The prep time includes time to make the pie crust. June

Makes: 4 generous servings
Prep Time: 1 hour
Bake Time: 45 to 50 minutes
Rest Time: 5 minutes after baking

Ingredients:

1 tablespoon grapeseed oil
1 large sweet onion, chopped
3/4 cup red bell pepper, diced

1/2 cup rice milk

---

5 large eggs
1/4 cup fresh parsley, chopped
1 teaspoon Mrs. Dash or other non-salt seasoning
1/2 teaspoon Seasoned Salt (see recipe in Mixes)
1/4 teaspoon ground pepper

---

4 slices turkey bacon, chopped

---

1 unbaked single Pie Crust (see recipe in Desserts)

Kitchen Tools:

9" pie pan

Measuring cups and spoons

12" skillet

Mixing bowl

Handheld mixer or whisk

Aluminum foil

Instructions:

1. Preheat oven to 325 degrees F (163 degrees C).
2. Heat the grapeseed oil in the skillet over medium heat, and add the onion and red pepper. Stir and sauté for 5 minutes, stirring often.
3. Remove from heat and stir in rice milk. Let cool for 5 minutes.
4. In a medium bowl, whisk eggs, parsley, non-salt seasoning, seasoned salt, and ground pepper. Whisk until well integrated and stir into vegetable mixture. Add the chopped bacon (no need to cook it if using turkey bacon).
5. Pour mixture into prepared pie crust. Using strips of aluminum foil, gently form foil over only the exposed pie crust edges, and press edges of foil onto the outside of the pie pan to secure the foil.
6. Bake 45 to 50 minutes, or until set in the middle and browned on top. When done, a knife inserted in the center will come out clean. Remove from oven, discard foil, and let rest for five minutes before serving.

Rice Crusted Scallion Quiche

This recipe came about one night when we needed a quick meal with what we had in the refrigerator. Making a standard pie crust was too time consuming, and since rice can be extremely versatile, adding seasonings and using it as a quiche base proved to be a good idea. The finished dish is high in protein, easy to make, colorful, and full of gentle flavor. If you choose brown rice instead of white rice, the result will be a more flavorful crust. June

Serves: 4
Prep Time: 30 minutes
Bake Time: 30 minutes
Rest Time: 5 minutes

Quiche Ingredients:

1 tablespoon sunflower oil
1 1/4 cups sliced scallions
1/2 cup diced red bell pepper

---

6 eggs
1/2 cup salt free Chicken Broth (see recipe in Mixes)
1 teaspoon dried dill weed
3/4 teaspoon salt

Crust Ingredients:

1 cup cooked rice, either brown or white
1/2 cup Daiya Cheddar Style Shreds cheese
1 tablespoon buttery spread, melted
1/2 teaspoon garlic powder
1/4 teaspoon Seasoned Salt (see recipe in Mixes)
1/8 teaspoon ground pepper

Kitchen Tools:

Cutting board and sharp knife

8" x 8" baking dish or pie pan

Small skillet

Small bowl

Measuring cups and spoons

Whisk or handheld mixer

Instructions:

1. Preheat oven to 350 degrees F (177 degrees C). Oil the baking dish and set aside.
2. Heat the oil in a small skillet and sauté the scallions and red pepper until soft, or about 5 minutes.
3. In a small bowl, beat together the eggs, chicken broth, dill weed, and salt. Stir into the vegetables and mix well. Set aside.
4. In a small bowl, mix together rice, Daiya cheese, buttery spread, garlic powder, seasoned salt, and pepper. Evenly press into the bottom and up the side of the baking dish to form a uniform crust.
5. Gently pour egg mixture over rice crust, and bake for 30 minutes or until a knife in the center of the dish comes out clean.
6. Remove from oven and let rest for 5 minutes before serving.

Spinach Leek Quiche

We find that a non-meat meal is a nice alternative, and this quiche is delicious. The dish was inspired by an Atkins low carb recipe and has been adapted to meet our dietary requirements. The time it takes to put this meal together is well worthwhile when you taste the end product. The prep time includes making the pie crust. June

Makes: 4 generous servings
Prep Time: 1 hour 15 minutes
Bake Time: 45 to 50 minutes
Rest Time: 5 minutes after baking

Ingredients:

1 1/2 lbs. leeks, white portion and 1" of the green (see step 2 on how to prepare)
1 tablespoon grapeseed oil

1/2 cup rice milk

---

1 10-oz. package frozen spinach, thawed and squeezed dry

---

4 large eggs
1/2 teaspoon Seasoned Salt (see recipe in Mixes)
1/4 teaspoon ground pepper

---

1 cup Daiya Mozzarella Style Shreds cheese, divided

---

1 unbaked single pie crust (see recipe in Desserts)

Kitchen Tools:

Medium skillet

9" pie pan

Measuring cups and spoons

Your favorite spatula

Mixing bowl

Handheld mixer or whisk

Aluminum foil

Instructions:

1. Preheat oven to 325 degrees F (163 degrees C).
2. To prepare leeks, cut about 1/2" off the bottom of the stalk. Cut the green tops off an inch above the white part, in the tender green area. Toss away the fibrous green leaves. Cut each leek in half the long way. Pull apart each layer of the leek and wash thoroughly in cold water in a large bowl. Leeks are grown in sandy soil and grit frequently finds its way into the layers. Change the water and wash leeks until there is no longer grit in the bottom of the bowl. Take your time and do a thorough job—your entire dish will end up in the garbage disposal if you bite down on grit. After thorough washing, slice leeks crosswise into thin slices.
3. Heat oil in skillet over medium heat and sauté leeks, stirring occasionally, for 5 to 6 minutes until softened. Remove from heat and stir in rice milk. Let cool for 5 minutes.
4. Meanwhile, thaw spinach and squeeze it dry.
5. In a medium bowl, whisk eggs, seasoned salt, and pepper. Switching to a fork, stir the spinach into the egg mixture, and combine with the leeks and rice milk. Mix well.
6. Sprinkle 3/4 cup Daiya cheese into the bottom of the pie shell. Add egg mixture and sprinkle the top with the remaining Daiya cheese.
7. Using strips of aluminum foil, gently form foil over only the exposed pie crust edges. Press edges of foil onto the outside of the pie pan to secure the foil.
8. Bake 45 to 50 minutes, or until set in the middle and browned on top. When done, a knife inserted in the center will come out clean. Remove from oven and let rest for 5 minutes before serving.

Variations:

Ham Option: Add 1 cup cubed ham with the spinach and egg mixture.

Eggs & Rice

Finding dishes my grandson can make quickly for himself for breakfast is a challenge, as is trying to ensure that he has a variety of foods to keep him satisfied. One morning we had leftover rice in the refrigerator, and I taught him how to make Eggs & Rice. He loved it and it's become a standard quick meal in our house. The buttery flavor of the fried rice and seasoned eggs just cooked until the whites are no longer runny, is a meal completed in ten minutes.

This meal is so simple it hardly needs a recipe, but we include it here as a reminder that a good meal doesn't need to be complicated. June

Serves: 2

Prep Time: 1 minute

Cooking Time: 10 minutes

Ingredients:

3 tablespoons buttery spread

2 cups cooked rice

1/2 teaspoon onion powder

1/4 teaspoon Seasoned Salt (see recipe in Mixes)

1/8 teaspoon black pepper

---

4 eggs

Kitchen Tools:

Large skillet

Measuring cups and spoons

Instructions:

1. Heat buttery spread in skillet on medium low heat and add the rice. Stir and fry for 1 minute to incorporate buttery spread.
2. Make 4 slight indentations in the rice with the back of a spoon, and gently break an egg into each hole. Sprinkle seasoned salt, onion powder, and ground pepper over rice, and cover with a tight fitting lid. Turn up heat to at least medium and, if it doesn't generate steam, add a tablespoon of water. Cook until whites are no longer liquid but yolks are still soft. Serve immediately.

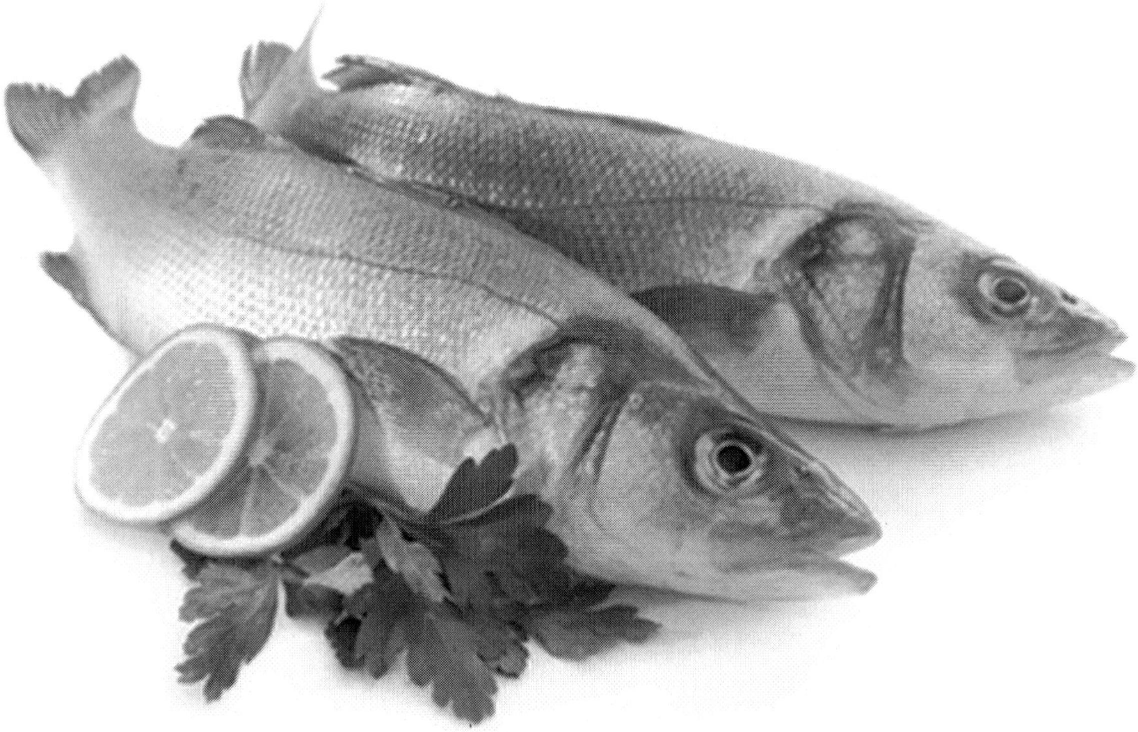

Fish & Seafood

When I was a child growing up in the land of 10,000 lakes, part of our regular diet was fresh water fish, which were cleaned and cooked within hours of catching. The best meals were the sunfish—small, broad, flat fish that were scaled and pan fried in butter, until each side was crisp. Even larger walleyes and northerns had that fresh, non-fishy taste that is rarely found in the ocean fish available to us in the East. The closest taste we found is the presently popular tilapia, and that's what we've specified in our recipes. However, if you prefer other types of fish, feel free to substitute whatever pleases your taste buds.

While the recipes in this section are few, the dishes are delicious. Be sure to try the Baked Fish Sticks and the Shrimp & Bacon Bake, which are kid endorsed.

Baked Fish Sticks

Most of us grew up with fish sticks served as a quick meal by our busy moms, or maybe in school cafeterias. In our house, it's called Deep Sea Chicken because it's the other white meat, but finding gluten free, soy free fish sticks without any forbidden ingredients is a real challenge. A search of every frozen food section always ended in disappointment.

The key to tasty fish sticks is in the crisp crumb coating. We've used a combination of dry gluten free bread crumbs, ground up vegetable chips, and potato chips. Other alternatives would be cracker crumbs or anything that would give you a crisp, tasty coating. The parchment paper keeps the fish from sticking and promotes even browning.

We always choose a mild tasting fish, so we've called for tilapia, but you can use whatever tickles your taste buds. Using different fish may allow you to experiment liberally with combining dried herbs in the coating mix. In any case, make it your own and enjoy fish sticks again! Kris

Serves: 4
Prep Time: 15 minutes
Bake Time: 15 to 20 minutes

Ingredients:

1 1/2 lbs. tilapia

---

1 egg well beaten

---

1 1/2 cups combination of dry gluten free bread crumbs and finely processed potato chips or other gluten-free chips
1 1/2 teaspoons Celery Salt (see recipe in Mixes)
3/4 teaspoon black pepper

Fresh lemon wedges

Kitchen Tools:

Baking sheet

Parchment paper

Cutting board and your favorite knife

2 shallow bowls

Instructions:

1. Preheat oven to 450 degrees F (232 degrees C). Cut parchment paper to fit baking sheet.
2. Cut the fish crosswise into 3/4" to 1" wide pieces while still partially frozen. Gently thaw and pour off any liquid.
3. In a shallow bowl, beat the egg until well broken down. Set aside.
4. Using a food processor, grind the bread crumbs and chips until finely processed. If the crumb mixture is too coarse, it will not stick to the fish. Combine crumbs, celery salt, and ground pepper in a second shallow bowl.
5. Using the one hand wet, one hand dry method, dip each fish stick in the egg. Place the fish in the crumb mixture and roll to coat, patting the crumbs into the fish. Place each piece of fish on the parchment paper without touching each other.
6. Bake until golden brown or 15 to 20 minutes. Serve with a squeeze of fresh lemon.

Shrimp & Bacon Bake

It was my turn to make dinner on a night in which I arrived home later than I intended. The stress was on to get dinner on the table at a reasonable hour, and I was desperate for inspiration as I rummaged through the freezer. A bag of frozen, cooked shrimp was just the answer! Not being much of a seafood lover, I looked at several cookbooks to see if I could make this shrimp dinner interesting. While each cookbook had wonderful ideas, I didn't have the ingredients needed for the recipes, nor did I have time to go to the grocery store. Another trip to the freezer turned up bacon and the inspiration was truly divine. I quickly threw some ingredients together and popped it in the oven, secretly hoping it wouldn't end up in the garbage disposal. What a surprise when this was one of the biggest successes of the week!

The beauty of this dish is in the simplicity of ingredients and easy preparation. This is a dish you can proudly serve your guests. Kris

Serves: 4

Prep Time: 15 minutes

Bake Time: 30 minutes

Ingredients:

1 to 1 1/2 lbs. shrimp, deveined, cooked, and shelled

1/2 cup olive oil

1/2 cup gluten free bread crumbs

1 teaspoon onion powder

1/2 teaspoon Celery Salt (see recipe in Mixes)

---

4 slices cooked, chopped bacon (if using turkey bacon, no need to cook)

Kitchen Tools:

8" x 11" baking dish

Measuring cups and spoons

Small bowl

Instructions:

1. Preheat oven to 400 degrees F (204 degrees C). Oil an 8" x 11" baking dish and set aside.
2. If shrimp is frozen, place in a strainer, and run under hot water for 30 seconds. Drain well. Place shrimp in baking dish and pour oil evenly over shrimp.
3. In a small bowl, mix bread crumbs, onion powder and celery salt. Sprinkle bread crumb mixture over shrimp and top with bacon.
4. Bake for 30 minutes and serve over your favorite pasta or rice.

Variations:

Lower Carb Option: If you're cutting carbs, eliminate the pasta or rice and serve over cooked spaghetti squash along with two vegetables.

Tilapia Option: Substitute tilapia filets for the shrimp and bake for 20 minutes until fish is flaky.

Tip: Turkey bacon is fully cooked so there's no need to pre-cook. There's a lot of conflicting reports on the healthful differences between turkey bacon and pork bacon, which all seem to revolve around which brands you choose. We simply prefer the taste of turkey bacon.

Baked Fish With Fresh Dill

The lemon and fresh dill make this recipe light and refreshing—and this is coming from someone who couldn't eat fish for 20 years. When I was pregnant with my second child, my first born would only eat tuna or banana sandwiches. The smell of tuna while I was pregnant was enough to put me off all fish for a very long time!

Fish is on our rotation plan, and this recipe was the result of my need to make a fish dish that had no fishy taste. We were thrilled to discover tilapia, a mild fish that doesn't have the heady, gamey flavor other fish has. If you think you hate fish, give this recipe a try, and if you love fish, you'll love the results. Kris

Serves: 4
Prep Time: 10 minutes
Bake Time: 15 minutes

Ingredients:

1/4 cup olive oil
1/4 cup chopped fresh dill or 1 tablespoon dried
3 tablespoons fresh squeezed lemon juice
2 tablespoons onion chopped
2 garlic cloves, minced
1/8 teaspoon pepper

---

1 to 1 1/2 lbs. tilapia fillets

Kitchen Tools:

Citrus juicer
Food processor
8" X 11" baking dish
Sharp chopping knife
Cutting board

Instructions:

1. Preheat oven to 425 degrees F (218 degrees C). Oil baking dish and set aside.
2. Place the olive oil, dill, lemon juice, onion, garlic, and pepper in the food processor. Process for 1 or 2 minutes until well blended.
3. Arrange tilapia fillets in the baking dish, and pour the oil and lemon mix over the fish. Bake for 12 to 15 minutes, until the fish flakes and pulls apart easily when probed with a fork. Serve immediately topped with liquids generated in baking.

Soups, Stews, & Casseroles

Soups and stews are often considered homey, comfort foods, that are filling and satisfying, like Beef and Mac Soup or Lentil Stew. Others can be served as an elegant first course, such as Creamed Carrot Soup or Cream of Celery Soup. Some recipes within these pages go together quickly and are ready in about an hour, while others require unattended simmering time or crockpot time, allowing you the freedom to do something else. All are made with fresh ingredients and herbs, which is reflected in the taste.

Most recipes call for our homemade beef, vegetable, or chicken broth, which is made without salt. If you use conventional broths, you will need to adjust the salt in the recipe.

These dishes freeze well for a grab and go lunch or a quick dinner. Served with fresh baked rolls, you have a complete meal.

Bacon Bean Soup

This soup is quick and easy to make, yet packed with vegetables and protein. The pungent flavor is perfectly offset by the fresh parsley and crumbled goat cheese. If your body can tolerate goat cheese, be sure to read the ingredients to ensure there's no cow's milk added. Serve with fresh hot rolls for a complete, satisfying meal. Kris

Makes: 9 cups
Prep Time: 30 minutes
Cook Time: 25 minutes

Ingredients:

2 tablespoons oil

---

2 yellow onions, chopped
2 carrots, diced
2 stalks celery, diced
1 small green pepper, diced
1 red bell pepper, diced

---

4 garlic cloves, minced

---

2 teaspoons Seasoned Salt (see recipe in Mixes)
2 teaspoons dried basil
1/2 teaspoon ground black pepper
1 bay leaf
3 1/2 cups salt free Chicken Broth (see recipe in Mixes)
1/2 cup coconut milk

---

1 15-oz. can Great Northern beans, rinsed and drained

---

1 15-oz. can garbanzo beans, rinsed and drained
1/2 cup salt free Chicken Broth

---

5 slices turkey bacon, chopped (There's no need to cook turkey bacon.)

1/2 cup fresh parsley, chopped

Crumbled goat cheese for garnish if tolerated (optional)

Kitchen Tools:

Measuring cups and spoons

Garlic press

Soup pot

Food processor

Cutting board and your favorite chopping knife

Instructions:

1. Heat the oil in the soup pot and add the onions, carrots, celery, green pepper, and red pepper. Stir and sauté for 10 minutes.
2. Add minced garlic and stir for 1 minute longer.
3. Stir in the seasoned salt, basil, pepper, bay leaf, chicken broth, and coconut milk. Heat to boiling.
4. Drain Great Northern beans, rinse, and drain again. Add to soup mix.
5. Drain garbanzo beans, rinse, and drain well. Place in a food processor with the 1/2 cup of chicken broth, and process until smooth. Stir into soup mix.
6. Chop bacon and add to soup. Simmer for 15 minutes until vegetables are tender.
7. Stir fresh parsley into soup and serve with crumbled goat cheese on each serving.

Beef & Mac Soup

Soups are especially warming on a cold winter day, and this soup is a delicious, hardy meal. The ingredients are minimal, but the effect is big and offers the perfect launch pad for your favorite herbs. This dish goes together easily for a quick meal. June

Serves: 6
Prep Time: 25 minutes
Cook Time: 30 minutes

Ingredients:

5 cups salt free Beef Broth (see recipe in Mixes)
1 cup salt free Vegetable Broth or Beef Broth (see recipes in Mixes)

---

2 1/2 cups celery, sliced
2 cups carrots, thinly sliced
1 large onion, coarsely chopped
2 tablespoons Italian Herb Mix (see recipe in Mixes)
1 tablespoon plus 1 teaspoon Seasoned Salt (see recipe in Mixes)
1 tablespoon basil
1 tablespoon onion powder
1/4 teaspoon allspice
1/4 teaspoon pepper
1 bay leaf

---

1 lb. ground beef

---

4 oz. gluten-free macaroni

Kitchen Tools:

Soup pot

Small skillet

2-quart saucepan

Measuring spoons

Cutting board

Your favorite slicing/chopping knife

Instructions:

1. Heat beef broth and vegetable broth in soup pot. Add the celery, carrots, onion, Italian herb mix, seasoned salt, basil, onion powder, allspice, pepper, and bay leaf. Simmer for 20 minutes.
2. While vegetables are simmering, fry ground beef in the skillet until browned. Drain off any fat that may have collected and discard it.
3. To cook macaroni, heat 1 quart or more of salted water in saucepan until boiling. Add macaroni, stirring to separate, and cook until barely tender. Drain immediately.
4. Stir ground beef and macaroni into vegetable mixture and bring to a boil. Simmer for 5 minutes. Remove bay leaf and serve.

Chicken Noodle Comfort Soup

Perhaps you have your own favorite chicken noodle soup recipe, or maybe you just wing it when you make soup. Go with what works for you, unless you're like me and always end up with enough soup to feed the Russian army. Unless I use a recipe, I can never get the proportions right, and that's why we're offering this recipe here. There are no weird ingredients, and the combination of the fresh vegetables, herbs, and broth gives you a classic soup that beats canned soup any day.

This recipe calls for precooked chicken, but if you have none on hand, allow extra time to cut chicken into 1/2" cubes and sauté until cooked. June

Serves: 6

Prep Time: 30 minutes

Cook Time: 20 minutes

Ingredients:

2 tablespoons oil

1 large sweet onion, chopped

3 stalks celery, diced

3 carrots, diced

1 cup green beans, cut into 1/2" pieces

1 purple topped turnip, peeled and diced

---

5 cups salt free Chicken Broth (see recipe in Mixes)

2 cups salt free Vegetable Broth (see recipe in Mixes)

2 teaspoons Seasoned Salt (see recipe in Mixes)

2 teaspoons Mrs. Dash Grilling Blends chicken flavor

1/2 teaspoon crushed basil

1/2 teaspoon ground celery seed

1/2 teaspoon rubbed sage

1/4 teaspoon turmeric

1/4 teaspoon allspice

1/8 teaspoon pepper

1 bay leaf

---

3 to 4 cups cooked, diced chicken

---

4 oz. uncooked gluten-free pasta of your choice

Kitchen Tools:

Soup pot

2-quart saucepan

Measuring spoons

Cutting board

Your favorite slicing/chopping knife

Instructions:

1. Heat the oil in your soup pot and add the onion, celery, carrots, green beans, and turnip. Sauté for 5 minutes, stirring often.
2. Add the chicken broth, vegetable broth, seasoned salt, Mrs. Dash, basil, celery seed, sage, turmeric, allspice, pepper, and bay leaf. Bring to a boil and simmer for 20 minutes until vegetables are soft. Stir in cooked chicken.
3. Meanwhile, bring water to a boil in a separate 2-quart saucepan, and cook the pasta according to packaged directions. Drain and add to individual bowls of soup when you serve. Gluten-free pasta will continue to soak up liquids in the soup, so it's best to keep it separate unless you don't mind if your leftover soup turns into stew.
4. Remove bay leaf and serve soup with fresh baked rolls.

Cream of Celery Soup

If you've ever had Cream of Celery soup out of a can, you should know up front this tastes nothing like the artificial taste you experienced. The first time I had homemade Cream of Celery Soup, it was as a long-time vegetarian. I was amazed that a "cream of" soup could taste so delicious and creamy, without any dairy or meat broth. We have duplicated the taste by using chicken broth as the base, which enhances the flavor of the vegetables.

The ingredients and seasonings in this recipe are simple and unsophisticated, but the taste is sensational and kid approved. We love it served with Pseudo Saltines (see recipe in Snacks). June

Makes: 8 cups
Prep Time: 60 minutes
Cook Time: 25 minutes

Ingredients:

2 tablespoons oil
4 cups celery, diced
3 cups potato, peeled and diced
1 large sweet onion, chopped

---

5 1/2 cups salt free Chicken Broth (see recipe in Mixes)

---

1 tablespoon Seasoned Salt (see recipe in Mixes)
1/2 teaspoon garlic powder
1/2 teaspoon black pepper

1/2 cup rice milk or coconut milk
1/4 cup plus 2 tablespoons cornstarch

1/2 cup fresh parsley, chopped

---

2 scallions, thinly sliced for garnish
10 slices cooked bacon, chopped for garnish

Kitchen Tools:

6-quart pan

Measuring cups and spoons

Cutting board

Chopping knife

Instructions:

1. Heat oil in pan on medium high heat, and add the celery, potatoes, and onion. Stir and sauté for a few minutes. Add the chicken broth and heat to boiling.
2. Add the seasoned salt, garlic powder, and pepper. When soup boils, reduce heat to low, and cook for 20 minutes until vegetables are soft.
3. Dissolve the cornstarch in the rice milk, and stir into the soup. Boil 1 minute, stirring constantly.
4. Remove from heat and transfer no more than three cups of soup into a blender. Remove the center of the blender cover, place a clean dry cloth over the hole to allow steam to escape, and turn the blender on low for 30 seconds. Pour into a large bowl and continue to puree soup in batches until the last batch. Process the last few cups for only a few seconds to allow the soup to have a bit of texture.
5. Reheat soup if necessary, and stir in the parsley. Serve with a sprinkle of sliced scallions and chopped bacon. Pseudo Saltines (see recipe in Snacks) make a delicious contrast.

Tip: Cut your "slicing and dicing" time in half by using the course-grating feature of your food processor.

Creamed Carrot Soup

We are always trying to get more vegetables into our diet in a satisfying way, and we give ourselves extra points if we incorporate a vegetable we don't normally use, such as turnips. Turnips can have a strong, distinctive taste, but when combined with the natural sweetness of carrots, the two exist in delicious harmony.

The original inspiration for this recipe was from the glutenfreeclub.com. We used the recipe as a launch pad and reworked the ingredients and process until it suited our taste and lifestyle. The end product is a soup with a light, naturally sweet flavor that comes primarily from the carrots. The color is vibrant, and this soup will be sure to be a hit as a first course or as the main course, served with gluten free rolls. Kris

Serves: 4
Prep Time: 30 minutes
Cook Time: 55 minutes

Ingredients:

1/4 cup oil
2 cups carrots, chopped
1 cup onions, chopped
1 cup purple topped turnip, chopped

---

5 cups salt free Chicken Broth or substitute up to 1 cup Vegetable Broth (see recipes in Mixes)
1 bay leaf
1 teaspoon Seasoned Salt (see recipe in Mixes)
Fresh ground black pepper to taste

---

2 1/2 cup cold rice milk
1/2 cup cornstarch

1/2 cup chopped fresh parsley

Kitchen Tools:

Cutting board and sharp knife

Food processor (optional)

Measuring cups and spoons

Your favorite vegetable peeler

6-quart cooking pot

Instructions:

1. In the cooking pot, heat oil and add carrots, onions, and turnip. Cook on medium low heat for 10 minutes, stirring occasionally.
2. Add the chicken or vegetable broth, bay leaf, seasoned salt, and pepper. Bring to a boil, cover, and gently simmer for 40 minutes until vegetables are tender. Remove bay leaf.
3. Stir cornstarch into cold rice milk until dissolved. Stirring constantly, add cornstarch mixture to soup and cook for 1 minute until thickened.
4. Remove from heat and transfer no more than 3 cups of soup to a blender. Remove the center of the blender cover, place a clean dry cloth over the hole to allow steam to escape, and turn the blender on low for 30 seconds. Pour into a large bowl. Continue to puree soup in batches until all soup has been processed.
5. Transfer soup back to the soup pot, and stir in chopped parsley. Gently heat again and serve hot.

Tip: Cut your "slicing and dicing" time in half by using the course-grating feature of your food processor.

Note: If you intend to freeze the soup, omit 1 3/4 cups of rice milk and add it upon thawing and reheating. Rice milk loses its integrity when frozen in combination with other ingredients.

Creamy Lentil Soup With A Kick

The inspiration for this recipe came from the internet, taking the best elements from various recipes and putting them together for an end product that is tasty, attractive, and easy to make. We were especially pleased with the result, because it required spices we wouldn't normally use.

Lentils are an inexpensive food, rich in protein, folate, thiamin, and iron. If you've never liked lentils or never even tried them, give this soup a chance, complete with the garnishes. Kris

Makes: 7 cups
Soak Time: 4 hours
Prep Time: 15 minutes
Cook Time: 30 minutes

Ingredients:

1 cup yellow or green lentils, washed and picked over

---

1 3/4 cups cold water
2 tablespoons turmeric
1 tablespoon salt

---

4 tablespoons oil
1 large onion, chopped

---

1 tablespoon garlic, minced

---

3 cups salt free Vegetable Broth (see recipe in Mixes)
1/2 cup coconut milk
2 tablespoons chili powder
2 teaspoons dried mint
2 teaspoons ground coriander

---

2 scallions for garnish, chopped
2 strips cooked bacon, crumbled or diced for garnish

Kitchen Tools:

Large cooking pot

Cutting board and sharp knife

10" skillet

Instructions:

1. Wash lentils in clear water, drain, and pick out foreign particles. Cover lentils with fresh clean water by 2". Let sit for at least 4 hours allowing lentils to expand.
2. Drain lentils, add 1 3/4 cups cold water, salt, and turmeric. Bring to a boil, turn heat down, and continue to simmer for 20 minutes until lentils are tender. If there is any excess liquid, strain. Return lentils to cooking pot and set aside.
3. In a 10" skillet, heat oil and fry onions on medium high heat until browned, stirring often. This is also known as caramelizing. Add garlic and cook for 1 minute, stirring constantly.
4. Stir onions and garlic into lentils, along with vegetable broth, coconut milk, chili powder, dried mint, and coriander. Heat and serve, topped with scallions and bacon.

Tip: We have heard for years that cooking some foods with salt, like beans and lentils, will make the food tough. Although you will see experts declare this emphatically as empirical truth, do your own test and you'll find this is one of the great food myths of all time. Cooking foods with salt distributes the salt evenly and elevates the flavor.

Six Layer Casserole

While rummaging through an old recipe box, I came across a yellowed index card with faded ink. It was for a layered casserole, which took me back to a remote farm in central Minnesota. My sister-in-law, Phyllis Kugler, came into my life when I needed her the most, and I will be forever grateful for the loving kindness and guidance she showed me. She was a farmer and a fabulous cook and baker. This was one of her dishes, and every time she made it, the house was filled with the myriad of delicious smells emanating from the oven that always elevated my appetite.

The liquid in the original recipe was tomato juice or V-8 Juice, and we've substituted chicken broth plus added a layer of celery. The end product is a delicious comfort food full of nutrition. June

Serves: 6

Prep Time: 35 minutes

Bake Time: 2 hours 15 minutes

Ingredients:

1 lb. lean ground beef

1/2 teaspoon Seasoned Salt (see recipe in Mixes)

---

1 large potato, sliced

1/2 cup uncooked rice, washed

1/4 teaspoon Seasoned Salt

---

2 cups sliced carrots

2 cups sliced celery

1/4 teaspoon Seasoned Salt

1 large onion, quartered and sliced

---

2 cups salt free Chicken Broth (see recipe in Mixes)

2 teaspoons non-salt seasoning such as Mrs. Dash

1 teaspoon Seasoned Salt

Kitchen Tools:

Medium skillet

2 1/2-quart casserole dish

Measuring cups and spoons

Cutting board

Your favorite knife

Instructions:

1. Oil the casserole dish and set aside. Preheat oven to 325 degrees F (163 degrees C).
2. In a dry skillet over medium heat, brown the ground beef with 1/2 teaspoon seasoned salt. Stir often. Remove from heat, drain, and discard excess fat.
3. Layer ingredients in the casserole dish in this order:
   - Sliced potato
   - Rice
   - 1/4 teaspoon Seasoned Salt
   - Ground beef
   - Carrots
   - Celery
   - 1/4 teaspoon Seasoned Salt
   - Onion
4. Heat chicken broth, and stir in non-salt seasoning and seasoned salt. Pour over vegetables, and bake uncovered for 1 hour 15 minutes.
5. Cover casserole and continue to bake for 1 more hour until vegetables are tender. Remove from oven and let rest for a few minutes before serving.

Note: The baking time is intended for a 2 1/2-quart casserole dish. If you choose a larger baking dish with more heating surface, you will need to adjust the baking time accordingly.

Crock Pot Beef Stew

Beef stew is one of those wonderful comfort foods that is especially good on a cold, winter day. I grew up on a farm in Minnesota and winter days there sometimes didn't get above the below zero mark. For those of us who now live in the South and have fewer cold days, using the crock pot is a great alternative to heating up the house with oven-baked dishes.

This recipe came out of a desire to give Kris less kitchen time and more time for herself. The stew goes together before I go to work, and is done when Kris comes home. There is nothing like the welcoming aroma of beef stew when you open the door. Serve this stew with freshly baked gluten-free rolls for a complete, satisfying meal. June

Serves: 6
Prep Time: 1 hour
Crock Pot Time: At least 6 hours

Ingredients:

2 lbs. stew meat, beef loin or round roast, fat removed and cut into 2" pieces

---

1/2 cup any gluten free flour mix
1 teaspoon Seasoned Salt (see recipe in Mixes)
1 teaspoon garlic powder
1/2 teaspoon pepper
1/2 teaspoon paprika

---

2 tablespoons oil

---

1 large onion quartered and cut into 1" pieces
1 lb. carrots, peeled and cut into 3/4" pieces
1 1/2 lbs. potatoes, washed and cut into 1" pieces
1 purple topped turnip, peeled and diced into 3/4" pieces

---

4 cups salt free Beef Broth (see recipe in Mixes)
1 teaspoon Mrs. Dash or other non-salt seasoning
1/2 teaspoon savory
1/4 teaspoon ground marjoram
2 large garlic cloves, minced
1 bay leaf

1/4 cup cold water
3 tablespoons cornstarch or arrowroot starch if freezing leftovers

Kitchen Tools:

Cutting board
Sharp knife
Crock Pot
Large nonstick skillet
Spatula for stirring and flipping meat
Measuring cups and spoons
Garlic press
1-quart saucepan
Gallon size resealable plastic bag

Instructions:

1. Place flour, seasoned salt, garlic powder, pepper, and paprika in a gallon size resealable bag. Add cut up beef, seal bag, and shake until beef is well coated.
2. Heat oil in large nonstick skillet and add meat. Brown over medium high heat until all sides are browned, turning occasionally. This should take about 15 minutes.
3. Meanwhile, oil sides and bottom of crock pot. Prepare the onion, carrots, potatoes, and turnip and place in bottom of crock pot.
4. When meat is browned, loosen meat and drippings with a spatula and add the beef broth. Add Mrs. Dash or equivalent, savory, marjoram, garlic, and bay leaf. Heat to boiling and pour over vegetables in crock pot.
5. Turn crock pot on high, cover, and cook for at least 6 hours or on low for 9 hours.
6. After stew is cooked, measure cold water and cornstarch into a 1-quart saucepan. Stir until cornstarch is dissolved. Stirring constantly, ladle a couple cups of liquid from the crock pot into the saucepan, and boil 1 minute. Combine gravy with vegetables and meat in crock pot. Adjust seasonings if necessary.
7. Serve in bowls with gluten-free rolls.

Variations:

Fresh Sage: Mince 2 tablespoons fresh sage leaves and add to beef broth in step 4.

Crock Pot Pork Over Potatoes

This recipe was a result of the need for a pork dish Kris would like. Pork is definitely not her favorite meat, but since it's part of our rotation plan of foods, I was determined to design a dish that didn't taste like pork. This was a winner in her mind because it made her taste buds sing. I love it because it is a no-fuss dish, designed to be simmered in the crock pot while I do something fun. The end result is tender, tasty, and perfect served over mashed potatoes or your favorite rice. June

Serves: 4 to 6
Prep Time: 30 minutes
Crock Pot Time: 4 to 6 hours or more

Ingredients:
3 or 4 lean pork chops, sliced into 1/2" strips
1 large onion quartered and sliced into 1/4" slices
1 bay leaf

---

1 1/2 cups rice milk
1/3 cup rice flour
1/2 cup salt free Beef Broth (see recipe in Mixes)
1 teaspoon Seasoned Salt (see recipe in Mixes)
1/2 teaspoon pepper
4 garlic cloves, minced

1/2 cup salt free Beef Broth
1/3 cup Bette Hagman's Modified GF Flour Mix (see recipe in Mixes)

Kitchen Tools:

1 1/2-quart saucepan

Cutting board

Sharp knife

Measuring cups and spoons

Crock pot

Small bowl

Instructions:

1. Slice the pork chops and put in bottom of crock pot. Add onion and bay leaf.
2. Stir rice flour into rice milk in the saucepan until there are no lumps. Add the beef broth, seasoned salt, pepper, and garlic. Heat over medium high heat, stirring constantly, until bubbling and slightly thickened. Pour liquid over pork chops and cover. Cook at least 6 hours on low or 4 hours on high.
3. Prepare the potatoes or rice while you finish step 4.
4. Remove the meat and put in a bowl. Ladle the liquid into a pan and bring to a boil. Measure 1/2 cup cold beef broth into a small bowl, add flour, and stir until dissolved. Pour flour combination into the hot liquid, stirring constantly, and continue to heat until thickened. Return meat to hot gravy and heat briefly. Serve over your choice of either mashed potatoes or your favorite rice.

Tip: If your job keeps you away from the house for long hours and your crock pot does not allow you to start and stop at a specific time, go to your local hardware store and get a programmable outlet. It's a neat little gadget that you plug into an outlet, and allows you to set time and day for starting and stopping whatever is plugged into that outlet.

Dilled Chicken Over Brown Rice

We are always in search of one-pot meals, and if it can be cooked in a crock pot, all the better. This recipe was engineered by combining our favorite flavors. There's nothing exotic or sophisticated about the ingredients, but the end product is flavorful, light and satisfying.

We've used our homemade chicken broth in this recipe, which has a rich, concentrated flavor. If your broth is light, you may want to add powdered broth, if you can find one that does not have forbidden ingredients. A second option is to add a couple teaspoons of non-salt seasoning. A third option is to heat twice as much light broth as you will need, and boil it down to half. That will intensify the flavor.

This dish can be served over mashed potatoes or white rice if you prefer, but the best choice is the slightly nutty flavor of long grain brown rice. June

Serves: 4

Prep Time: 45 minutes

Crock Pot Time: 4 hours

Ingredients:

2 to 3 lbs. boneless chicken breasts
2 tablespoons oil

---

1 yellow onion quartered and sliced
3 cups celery, cut diagonally in 1/2" pieces

---

1 cup salt free Chicken Broth (see recipe in Mixes)
1/2 cup rice flour
2 tablespoons dried dill weed
1 teaspoon ground mustard
1 teaspoon Seasoned Salt (see recipe in Mixes)
1/2 teaspoon pepper

---

1 1/2 cups salt free Chicken Broth or combination of Vegetable Broth (see recipes in Mixes)

Cooked long grain brown rice

Kitchen Tools:

Measuring cups and spoons

Skillet

Crock Pot

Instructions:

1. Heat oil in the skillet and cook the chicken breasts until browned.
2. While chicken is browning, prepare the onion and celery, and put in the bottom of the crock pot.
3. In a small bowl, stir together the chicken broth, flour, dill weed, ground mustard, seasoned salt, and pepper until flour is dissolved.
4. When chicken is browned, remove from skillet and place on top of the vegetables in the crock pot.
5. Heat 1 1/2 cups broth in the skillet and stir to loosen and incorporate any browned bits of chicken. Stirring constantly, pour broth and flour mixture into skillet and boil 1 minute.
6. Pour broth mixture over chicken and cover crock pot. Cook on high for 4 hours.
7. Serve over cooked brown rice.

Italian Vegetable Soup

We particularly like Italian food, but neither Kris nor I can have tomatoes, which is a huge part of the satisfaction of Italian food. The next best thing is pesto, and this soup has just such a base. You can use our pesto recipe in the Sauces section, or a prepared pesto if you're short on time. The combination of vegetables, chicken, and seasonings make this a great cold weather soup, and a complete meal when served with your favorite gluten-free rolls. As with all our recipes, feel free to make it your own by using different vegetables or adjust the seasonings to your taste. June

Serves: 6 to 8
Prep Time: 40 minutes
Cook Time: 20 minutes

Ingredients:
1 lb. chicken breasts, cut into 1" pieces
4 cups salt free Chicken Broth (see recipe in Mixes)

---

1 1/2 cups salt free Vegetable Broth (see recipe in Mixes)
1/2 cup prepared Pesto Sauce (see recipe in Sauces)
2 teaspoons salt
1/2 teaspoon dried oregano
1/2 teaspoon dried savory
1 teaspoon dried basil
5 drops SweetLeaf liquid stevia

---

1 cup fresh green beans, cut into 1/2" lengths
1/2 cup onion, chopped
4 medium carrots, peeled and cut into 1/4" slices
1 purple top turnip, peeled and cut into 3/4" cubes
2 stalks celery, cut in 1/4" slices
4 garlic cloves, minced

---

1 medium zucchini, quartered and sliced

2/3 cup chopped fresh parsley

Kitchen Tools:

4 1/2-quart saucepan

Cutting board and your favorite sharp knife

Measuring cups and spoons

Small bowl

Instructions:

1. Boil chicken and chicken broth together until chicken is tender, about 5 minutes. When done, transfer the chicken to a small bowl with a slotted spoon and set aside.
2. Return the broth to boiling and add the vegetable broth, pesto sauce, salt, basil, oregano, savory, and stevia.
3. When boiling once again, add the green beans, onion, carrots, turnip, celery, and garlic. Cover and boil for 8 minutes, until vegetables are almost tender.
4. Add the zucchini and chicken, and boil for 3 minutes until all vegetables are tender.
5. Stir in parsley and serve hot.

Lentil Stew

Lentils are an inexpensive food that is rich with nutrients. Lentils, by themselves, have a rather bland taste that will take on the flavor of whatever herbs and meats are combined with them. This recipe calls for Kitchen Bouquet Browning & Seasoning Sauce, found in most grocery stores. It is a condensed brown sauce used to season and add coloring. The customer service agent for the distributor assured me the ingredients are gluten and soy free.

There are so many possibilities of pleasing flavors to combine with lentils, and we put together the flavors we like the most, but feel free to exclude anything you don't like and add ingredients you prefer. June

Makes: Approximately 18 cups
Soak Time: 4 to 8 hours
Prep Time: 55 minutes
Cook Time: 2 hours

Ingredients:

1 3/4 cups lentils

---

3 1/2 cups salt free Beef Broth (see recipe in Mixes)
2 1/2 cups cold water
3 1/2 oz. turkey bacon or smoked pork, chopped
1 1/2 cups carrots, diced
1 1/2 cups celery, sliced
1 zucchini, diced
1 large onion, chopped
1 potato, peeled and diced
2 tablespoons olive oil
2 garlic cloves, minced

---

1 tablespoon Seasoned Salt (see recipe in Mixes)
2 bay leaves
1/2 teaspoon ground pepper

---

1 tablespoon Kitchen Bouquet Browning & Seasoning Sauce

Kitchen Tools:

Large cooking pot

Cutting board and sharp knife

Stirring spoon

Instructions:

1. Wash lentils in cold water, drain, and pick out foreign particles as well as any wrinkled lentils. Rinse again in water and drain. Cover lentils by 2" with fresh, clean water. Let sit for at least 4 hours or overnight, allowing lentils to expand.
2. Drain lentils and add enough water to cover. Boil for 2 minutes and drain the greyed water. Add beef broth, cold water, bacon, carrots, celery, zucchini, onion, potato, olive oil, and garlic.
3. Stir in the seasoned salt, bay leaves, and pepper. Return to a boil and turn heat down to simmer. Set timer for 2 hours, stirring occasionally.
4. Add the Kitchen Bouquet and stir to combine. Serve hot with Pseudo Saltines (see recipe in Snacks) or fresh baked rolls.

Note: This dish freezes well.

Quinoa Sausage Soup

Quinoa is fabulously versatile and nutritious, and takes on the flavor of whatever you combine with it. For this dish, the sausage is the dominant flavor, and the type you choose will determine the taste of your soup. We chose a mild Italian sausage, which gives it a slightly spicy flavor, but feel free to make other choices.

Because quinoa will continue to expand in liquid, we suggest scooping a quantity of cooked quinoa into the bottom of each bowl, and pour the soup over it just before serving. This soup is hearty, delicious, and full of protein. Kris

Serves: 4

Prep Time: 30 minutes

Cook Time: 40 minutes

Ingredients:

3/4 lb. mild Italian sausage

---

2 tablespoons oil

---

2 cups sweet onions, chopped

2 cups celery, sliced

2 cups carrots, sliced

---

3 garlic cloves, minced

---

3 cups salt free Beef Broth (see recipe in Mixes)

1 cup salt free Vegetable Broth (see recipe in Mixes)

1 bay leaf

1 teaspoon Seasoned Salt (see recipe in Mixes)

1 teaspoon Herbes De Provence

1/4 teaspoon black pepper

1/2 cup raw quinoa

3/4 cup water

1/4 teaspoon salt

Kitchen Tools:

Medium skillet

Soup pot

1 1/2-quart saucepan

Measuring spoons

Garlic press

Instructions:

1. In a medium skillet, brown sausage and drain off and discard any excess fat. Set aside.
2. Heat oil over medium heat in the soup pot. Add the onion, carrots, and celery. Stir and sauté for 5 minutes.
3. Add garlic and stir and cook for 1 additional minute.
4. Add beef broth, vegetable broth, bay leaf, seasoned salt, Herbes De Provence, pepper, and sausage. Reduce heat to low and simmer for 15 minutes.
5. While soup is simmering, rinse quinoa at least three times and drain through a splatter screen. In the smaller saucepan, combine 3/4 cup water with the quinoa and salt. Heat to boiling, cover, reduce heat to low, and simmer for 15 to 20 minutes until water is absorbed. Watch it closely in the last 10 minutes to ensure the quinoa doesn't burn. Fluff quinoa and set aside.
6. When onions, carrots, and celery are tender, remove bay leaf. To serve, place 1/3 cup cooked quinoa in the bottom of the soup bowl. Top with 1 1/2 cups of soup and serve immediately. Store any leftover soup and quinoa separately, as quinoa continues to expand in liquid.

Ragout de Porc

The warmth and smell of a stew slowly cooking is irresistible on cold winter days, and this stew is as tasty as its aroma. This dish has a brief prep period in a skillet, but the majority of the cooking is done in a crock pot, and the fact that you can fix it and forget it for four hours is a bonus. Use any mixed vegetable combination that works for you. The rice is cooked separately, and becomes the base for the stew when served. June

Serves: 4
Prep Time: 25 minutes
Crock Pot Time: 4 hours

Ingredients:

1 tablespoon oil
1 1/2 lbs. pork tenderloin, cut into 1" cubes

---

1 large sweet onion, chopped
2 stalks celery, sliced
1 1/2 teaspoons Seasoned Salt (see recipe in Mixes)
1/2 teaspoon dried basil
1/2 teaspoon Herbes De Provence
1/2 teaspoon ground black pepper
1/4 teaspoon dried rosemary

---

3 tablespoons Bette Hagman's Featherlight Flour Mix (see recipe in Mixes)
1 cup cold salt free Beef Broth (see recipe in Mixes)
8 oz. (or more) frozen mixed vegetables

---

1 package (6.2 oz.) long grain and wild rice

Kitchen Tools:

Crock Pot

Skillet

Measuring cups and spoons

Instructions:

1. Heat oil in skillet over medium high heat and, when hot, add pork. Stir and sear meat for a few minutes. Add onion, celery, seasoned salt, basil, Herbes De Provence, pepper, and rosemary. Cook, stirring often until vegetables are soft, approximately 8 minutes. Transfer pork mixture to crock pot.
2. Stir flour into beef broth until dissolved, and pour into crock pot along with the mixed vegetables. Stir to distribute ingredients.
3. Cover crock pot and cook on low for 4 hours.
4. Toward end of cooking time, prepare rice according to packaged directions. Depending on the brand and type of rice, allow 20 to 45 minutes for rice to cook. Fluff rice, spoon a portion into each bowl, and serve stew over rice.

Tomato-less Chili

There isn't ***less*** *tomato in this recipe; there isn't* ***any*** *tomato at all, so the name is a misnomer (or would that be misnamer?) This recipe was designed to get more beans and vegetables into our diet. We missed the tomato-based chili we had always known but could no longer have, so we consulted various recipes, and then took the best from all of them, with a wonderfully flavorful result.*

If you are unable to find ground pork, a meatloaf mixture of ground pork, beef and veal will work nicely. June

Serves: 6

Prep Time: 40 minutes

Cook Time: 35 to 45 minutes

Ingredients:

1/2 lb. ground pork

1/2 lb. ground beef

1 large red onion, diced

---

5 garlic cloves, minced

---

1 15-oz. can pinto beans, drained and rinsed

1 15-oz. can black beans, drained and rinsed

---

3 carrots, diced in 1/2" pieces

3 stalks celery, diced in 1/2" pieces

2 cups salt free Beef Broth (see recipe in Mixes)

2 tablespoons chili powder

1 teaspoon ground cumin

1 teaspoon Seasoned Salt (see recipe in Mixes)

---

1 tablespoon cornstarch

1/2 cup cold water

Kitchen Tools:

Large skillet or 6 quart cooking pot

Measuring cups and spoons

Instructions:

1. In a skillet or cooking pot, cook the ground beef, pork, and onion on medium high heat until browned. Drain and discard any fat that may be left.
2. Add garlic and cook for 1 minute, stirring constantly.
3. Drain and rinse beans to remove gas-causing agents. Add to meat mixture.
4. Add carrots, celery, beef broth, chili powder, cumin, and seasoned salt. Bring to a boil, cover, and simmer for 35 to 45 minutes until vegetables are tender, stirring occasionally.
5. In a cup, stir cornstarch into cold water until dissolved. Stirring constantly, pour into chili and bring to a boil. Gently cook for 1 minute.
6. Serve in bowls with Cornbread (see recipe in Breads) or Veggie Biscuits (see recipe in Muffins).

Variations:

Beanless Option: If beans are difficult for you to digest, eliminate the beans and serve over cooked quinoa.

Chicken Rice Bake

It was a late Sunday afternoon and we had no clue what to fix for dinner. I remembered a recipe in a dusty old recipe box, that called for chicken baked on a bed of rice, with canned creamed soup and Lipton Onion soup mix. It was totally delicious, easy to make, and wonderfully inexpensive. Unfortunately, the soups which constituted the majority of the flavor have become forbidden foods for us, but we designed a great recipe for Onion Soup & Dip Mix, which became the base for this dish. This version comes really close to the original taste, with no fuss and the simplest of ingredients. Enjoy this casserole with your favorite green vegetables. June

Serves: 6

Prep Time: 10 minutes

Bake Time: 1 hour 15 minutes

Ingredients:

1 to 2 lbs. boneless chicken cutlets

1/2 to 3/4 teaspoon non-salt garlic and herb seasoning

1/3 cup Onion Soup & Dip Mix (see recipe in Mixes)

2 cups salt free Chicken Broth (see recipe in Mixes)

2 cups thinly sliced celery

---

1 cup long grain white or brown rice, washed

Kitchen Tools:

9" x 13" baking dish

1 1/2-quart saucepan

Measuring cups

Aluminum foil

Instructions:

1. Preheat oven to 350 degrees F (177 degrees C). Oil baking dish and set aside.
2. Combine onion soup and dip mix, chicken broth, and celery in a saucepan. Heat to boiling. Stir in the washed rice and pour into baking dish.
3. Position chicken on rice mixture, sprinkle chicken with non-salt seasoning, cover with foil, and bake for 1 hour 15 minutes.

Tip: You can easily prep this dish in the morning or the night before. Thaw out chicken cutlets and refrigerate. Wash rice in saucepan, drain and stir in onion soup and dip mix, chicken broth, and celery. Refrigerate and, when ready to bake, heat broth mixture to boiling. Pour into baking dish and continue with step 3.

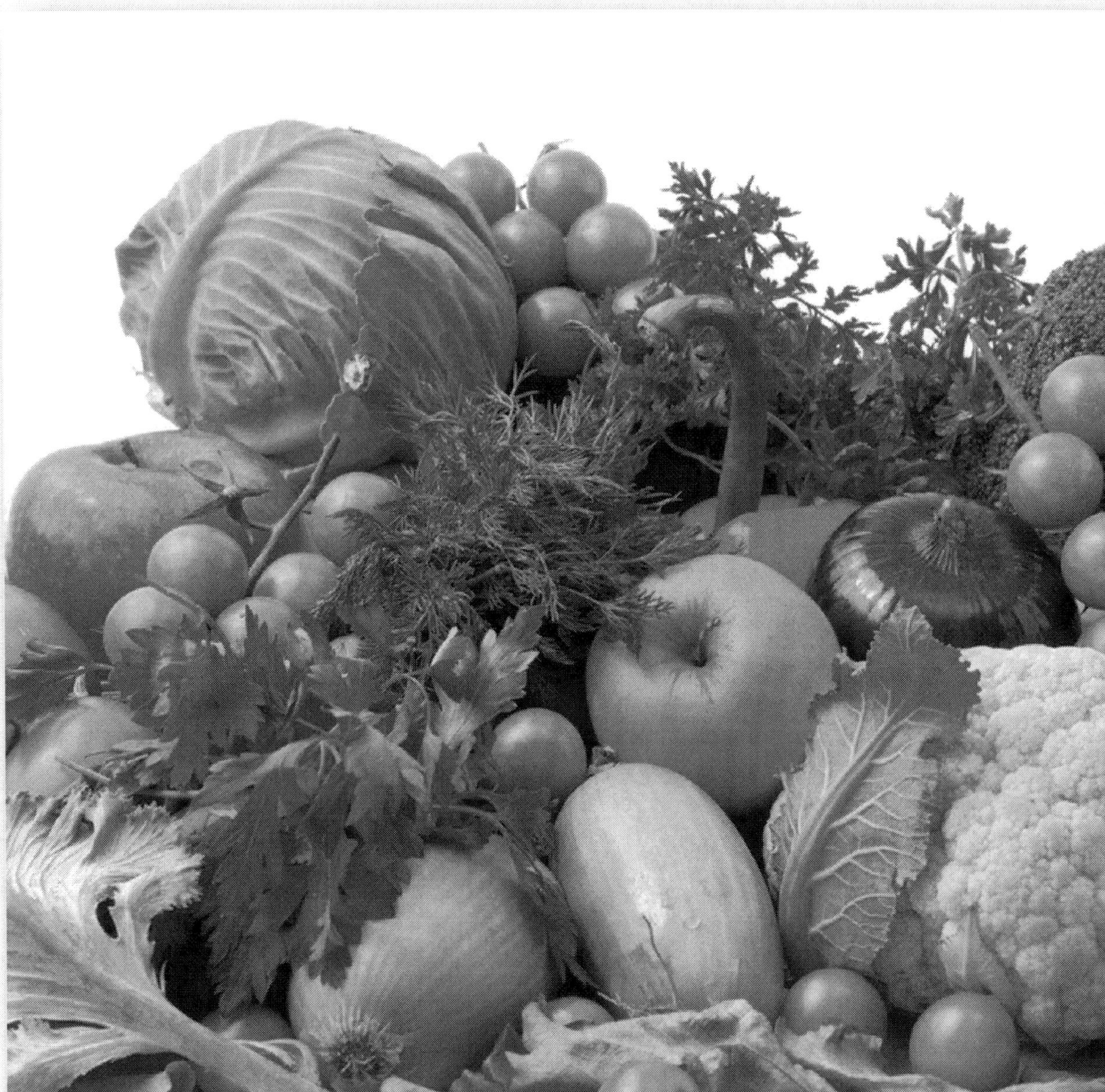

VEGETABLES

One of the drawbacks to most of the cookbooks we have seen, is the limited number of creative vegetable recipes in each. We understand the importance of vegetables in our diet, and strive to serve two veggies with each meal. We took on the challenge to present as many flavorful vegetable recipes as possible in this cookbook.

Within this section, you will find a great deal of variety, from Baked Asparagus to Zucchini Fritters, Mashed Parsnips, Carrots & Sweet Potatoes to Potato Latkas. If you try no other recipe, do make the Quinoa Tabbouleh, which has gotten rave reviews from everyone who has tried it.

Broccoli Cauliflower Hollandaise

This recipe was the result of a desire to find a delicious way to serve a vegetable none of us particularly like: cauliflower. By itself, cauliflower is pretty boring, but mashed into potatoes or served with broccoli and hollandaise gives it new respect.

While Hollandaise is incredibly easy to make, it cannot be rushed. It's essential to start out with very cold buttery spread, stir constantly, and keep the temperature at low.

Hollandaise transforms almost any vegetable into an elegant dish. The buttery lemon flavor is a natural for any greens, broccoli, cauliflower, or eggs. June

Serves: 4

Prep Time: 10 minutes

Cook Time: 15 minutes

Ingredients:

1/2 lb. fresh cauliflower

1/2 lb. fresh broccoli

Sauce Ingredients:

2 egg yolks

3 tablespoons fresh lemon juice

1/4 teaspoon salt

1/4 teaspoon onion powder

1/2 cup very cold buttery spread

Kitchen Tools:

Cutting board

Your favorite vegetable knife

Small saucepan

2 1/2-quart saucepan

Vegetable steamer

Measuring spoons and cups

Citrus juicer

Whisk

Instructions:

1. Rinse broccoli and cauliflower and drain well. Cut flowerets into uniform sizes and steam until almost tender. Keep in mind, vegetables will continue to cook after you shut off the heat. Keep them warm.
2. While vegetables are cooking, put egg yolks, lemon juice, salt, and onion powder into the small saucepan. Whisk to mix well.
3. Add half the cold buttery spread and turn the heat on low (seriously, don't try to rush this process by turning up the heat). Whisking constantly, heat gently to melt the butter, and give the egg yolks time to cook and thicken the sauce.
4. Add the remainder of the cold buttery spread and continue whisking until the buttery spread is melted and sauce is thick. If you've followed the directions to this point, the buttery spread is properly melted, and the sauce is not thick, turn up the heat just a tad to cook egg yolks. Whisk constantly until sauce is thick. Remove from heat.
5. Serve vegetables immediately with sauce over.

Note: If sauce separates, slowly stir in 1 teaspoon water, heating on low. Store any leftover hollandaise in the refrigerator. To reuse, stir a tablespoon of boiling water into leftover hollandaise and serve. Do not microwave sauce.

Variations:

Dill Option: Add 2 tablespoons fresh minced dill to finished sauce.

Italian Green Beans

It was Labor Day, and we had been out shopping all afternoon in our favorite health food stores, drooling over foods I couldn't have. I hadn't had lunch, and my nutritional reserves were in the negative numbers. We were in a rush to make dinner, tired of the same old vegetables the same old way, and that's how this recipe came about. I incorporated our favorite flavors, cooked together until the beans were just tender and bright green. The end result was a great accompaniment to Chicken Piccata. Kris

Serves: 4
Prep Time: 20 minutes
Cook Time: 8 minutes

Ingredients:

3/4 lb. fresh green beans or good quality frozen

---

2 tablespoons olive oil
1/4 cup coarsely chopped onions
1/2 teaspoon dried basil
1/2 teaspoon Seasoned Salt (see recipe in Mixes)

---

1 garlic clove, minced

Kitchen Tools:

Small nonstick skillet or nonstick saucepan
Wooden spoon
Cover for skillet or saucepan
Garlic press

Instructions:

1. Wash green beans, drain, and cut into 1 1/2" pieces.
2. Heat oil over medium heat in the skillet or saucepan. Add green beans, onions, basil, and seasoned salt. Stir to incorporate seasonings and oil.
3. Cook, stirring often for 4 minutes. Add a couple tablespoons of water, cover, and steam for 2 minutes until green beans are just tender.
4. Add the garlic and stir, continuing to cook for 1 minute. Shut off heat and serve immediately. If not serving immediately, know that the green beans will continue to cook a bit even with the heat off.

Variations:

Lemon Option: Just before serving, stir in 1 tablespoon of fresh lemon juice.

Tangy Cucumber Dill Salad

Harbin Farms has a farm stand a block away from our house, and their fresh cucumbers taste like I remember them from the farm when I was a kid. There is a refreshing element about cucumber that you just can't get from any other vegetable. The crisp, mild flavor lends itself to fresh lemon juice enhanced by dill, and that was the inspiration for this recipe. The beauty of this recipe is the simplicity of the ingredients that make it tangy and refreshing, plus being beautiful—a combination that can't be beat. Kris

Serves: 4
Prep Time: 20 minutes
Cooling Time: 30 minutes or more

Ingredients:

3 cups cucumbers, peeled, seeded and sliced in 1/4" slices
3 tablespoons chopped pimento

1/4 cup fresh lemon juice
1 1/2 teaspoons Dill Seasoning (see recipe in Mixes)
3/4 teaspoon salt

Kitchen Tools:

Cutting board and your favorite knife
Vegetable peeler
Medium bowl
Small bowl
Citrus juicer
Measuring cups and spoons

Instructions:

1. Prepare cucumber and combine with pimento in a medium bowl.
2. In a small bowl, mix together the lemon juice, dill seasoning, and salt.
3. Pour lemon mixture into cucumbers and stir well. The lemon juice will encourage some of the moisture out of the cucumber, and the flavors will blend together. Refrigerate for at least 30 minutes or longer, and serve chilled.

Variations:

Less Tang and More Sweet: If the taste is a bit too tangy for you, experiment with the amount of lemon juice and add 1 drop of liquid stevia at a time to the lemon juice, salt and dill seasoning mixture, until you reach the taste you want.

Perfect Protein Salad

The inspiration for this dish came from the Sugar Solution Cookbook by the Editors of Prevention Magazine with Ann Fittante, copyright 2006, published by Rodale, Inc. This was one of the first cookbooks we bought in our early quest for better health through regulating blood sugar naturally—just one direction in our research process. The original recipe called for ingredients we could not have, such as couscous, capers, and feta cheese. We've substituted quinoa, eliminated some ingredients, and added others to give us the taste we wanted. The quinoa is a complete protein, and the combined taste is out of this world. It's best if you can refrigerate overnight, but will also be delicious if served immediately. June

Makes: 6 cups
Prep Time: 50 minutes
Cook Time: 25 minutes
Cooling Time: 30 minutes

Ingredients:
1 cup uncooked quinoa

---

1 1/4 cups cold water
1/2 teaspoon salt

---

1 can red kidney beans, rinsed and drained
1 1/4 cups cucumber, peeled, seeded and chopped (1 medium)
1/2 cup green bell pepper, diced
3/4 cup red bell pepper, diced
1/2 cup red onion, finely chopped
1/3 to 1/2 cup chopped fresh dill
2 tablespoons vinegar free green olives, drained and chopped

3/4 cup lemon juice (approximately 2 large lemons)
1/2 cup light olive oil
1 1/4 teaspoons Seasoned Salt (see recipe in Mixes)

1/4 teaspoon freshly ground black pepper

Sliced ripe avocado

Kitchen Tools:

1-quart saucepan

Citrus juicer

Measuring cups and spoons

Medium bowl

Small bowl

Small whisk

Splatter screen

Instructions:

1. Measure quinoa into saucepan, and fill pan with cold water. Gently swish the quinoa around to wash the bitter coating off the grain. Using a splatter screen held firmly over the pan, drain the water. Repeat this process two more times.
2. Measure cold water and salt into pan with the quinoa, and heat on high until water boils. Immediately turn heat down to very low, cover, and cook for 15 to 20 minutes. Watch the last few minutes to ensure quinoa doesn't burn. Remove from heat and, while still covered, allow to rest for another 5 minutes. Fluff quinoa with a fork and spread out on a large plate or baking sheet. Cool in the refrigerator for 30 minutes or longer unrefrigerated.
3. Meanwhile, drain and rinse the kidney beans and put in the medium bowl. Add the prepared cucumber, green pepper, red pepper, red onion, dill, and olives.
4. In the small bowl, whisk together the lemon juice, olive oil, seasoned salt, and pepper. Pour over vegetables. Add the cooled quinoa and stir to combine. Chill or serve immediately with sliced avocado.

Potato Latkas

Potato Latkas, also known as potato pancakes, is a traditional Jewish dish served during Hanukkah. I'm grateful we can have them any time of the year, as they are absolutely delicious and a nice change from mashed or baked potatoes. Either fry them in batches and keep them warm in the oven, or use a large griddle or electric skillet to cut down on cooking time. Potato latkas are a great accompaniment to eggs, hamburgers, or ham. June

Serves: 4
Prep Time: 30 minutes
Cook Time: 30 minutes

Ingredients:

2 cups finely shredded raw potatoes, approximately 1 large (no need to peel it)

1/2 cup grated onion

---

1 egg, beaten
1/2 cup Bette Hagman's Modified GF Flour Mix (see recipe in Mixes)
1 teaspoon Baking Powder (see recipe in Mixes)
1 teaspoon salt
1/2 teaspoon pepper

Oil for frying

Kitchen Tools:

Medium bowl
Small bowl
Measuring cups and spoons
Handheld mixer of whisk
Food processor or grater
Large skillet or griddle

Instructions:

1. Grate potatoes and immediately place them in cold water for up to 5 minutes. Drain well in a strainer. Handful by handful, squeeze out as much moisture as possible and place in a bowl. Squeeze or press excess moisture out of the grated onion and add to the potatoes.
2. In a small bowl, beat eggs, flour, baking powder, salt, and pepper. Mixture will be thick. Add the potatoes and onion and mix well. Let sit for 5 to 10 minutes.
3. Heat a couple tablespoons of oil in the skillet or griddle over medium heat until hot. Stir mixture to reincorporate the liquid that has leached out, and drop large tablespoons of the potato mixture onto the hot oil. Using a spatula, flatten each latka, flip over, and flatten the second side of each latka to less than 1/4". Brown for 3 or 4 minutes per side and then remove to drain on a paper towel.
4. Serve warm, plain, or topped with buttery spread.

Quinoa Tabbouleh

It was a Saturday afternoon and Kris, Jonathan, and I were shopping at a market in Columbia, Maryland called Mom's Organic Market. It was our first time in the store, and as we checked out the various foods and products, we were offered samples to taste. Quinoa Tabbouleh was one of the dishes offered, and we didn't need more than one bite to know we had found a new favorite food.

Quinoa is a versatile, ancient grain, cultivated in the South American Andes since at least 3000 BC. It's high in protein, calcium, and iron, as well as a pretty good source of several B vitamins and vitamin E. It contains a perfect balance of all nine essential amino acids needed for tissue development, which makes it a perfect protein.

This recipe lends itself to any raw vegetables you would like to use. Proportions can be changed, as well as the amount of oil and lemon juice to suit your taste. This salad is best if it's allowed to marinate for 8 or more hours, but will be tasty if eaten immediately. June

Serves: 6

Prep Time: 1 hour 40 minutes

Cook Time: 20 minutes

Ingredients:

1 cup quinoa

1 1/4 cups water

---

2 cups red and yellow peppers, seeded, cut into 3/8" pieces

3 stalks celery, cut into 3/8" pieces

2 carrots shredded

1 cup minced scallion (1 bunch) or 2 tablespoons onion powder

1 cup fresh parsley, chopped (1 bunch)

1 large cucumber, seeded and diced

1/4 to 1/2 cup fresh lemon juice (1 1/2 lemons) or more to taste

1/4 cup extra virgin olive oil or any light tasting oil

1 1/2 teaspoons Seasoned Salt (see recipe in Mixes) or less to taste

Fresh ground black or colored pepper

Kitchen Tools:

Large bowl

Sharp knife

Your favorite cutting board

Citrus juicer

Measuring cups and spoons

Large baking sheet

Splatter screen

Instructions:

1. Rinse quinoa in cold water and drain through splatter screen to remove the bitter coating. Repeat this process two more times. To cook the quinoa, add 1 1/4 cups cold water and heat to boiling. Reduce heat to low, cover, and simmer for 15 to 20 minutes or until water is absorbed. Check to ensure the quinoa doesn't burn in the last few minutes. Remove from heat and let rest, still covered, for another 5 minutes.
2. Fluff quinoa and spread out on a large baking sheet to cool for an hour.
3. Meanwhile, prepare the vegetables and stir together in a large bowl. Add the cooled quinoa and mix.
4. In a small bowl, whisk together the lemon juice, olive oil, seasoned salt, and pepper. Add to vegetables and stir until thoroughly combined.
5. This salad is best if refrigerated for at least a couple of hours or overnight before serving, but also good if eaten immediately.

Note: You may need to add more oil, lemon, or seasonings to get it just the way your taste buds like it. I (Kris) like a modest amount of lemon juice, while my mother delights in heavy lemon flavor. Do whatever works for you.

Variations:

Less Raw Vegetables: If your body has issues with certain raw vegetables, sauté broccoli, cauliflower, and asparagus in buttery spread until barely cooked but still crisp. Turn off heat, add a couple cloves of minced garlic, and stir to mix well. Set aside and cool before adding to the rest of the Tabbouleh ingredients.

Raw Onion Alternative: If your body doesn't do well with raw onions but you still like the onion flavor, finely chop a large red or white onion and add it to the quinoa before cooking. The flavor will permeate the quinoa but not overwhelm it. Another option is to stir onion powder into lemon juice.

Scalloped Carrots & Turnips

The inspiration for this recipe was a childhood memory of scalloped carrots my mother made, using the sweet carrots out of our garden, and milk fresh from our cows. She never wrote down the recipe, so I had to go to the internet for guidance. I found an innovative recipe combining carrots and turnips on www.cooks.com, a great website with a terrific recipe base. We've changed the seasonings, added chicken broth, and made it dairy free and gluten free. If you've never had turnips, let this be your introduction. This dish passed the kid test! June

Serves: 6
Prep Time: 40 minutes
Bake Time: 30 minutes

Ingredients:

2 cups purple top turnips, cut into 1/2" pieces
1 1/2 cups carrots sliced in 3/8" slices
1 teaspoon salt

---

3 tablespoons buttery spread or olive oil
3 tablespoons any gluten free flour mix

---

1 cup rice milk
1/2 cup salt free Chicken Broth (see recipe in Mixes)
1/2 teaspoon salt
1/2 teaspoon onion powder
2 teaspoons Dill Seasoning (see recipe in Mixes)

1/3 cup gluten free bread crumbs or crushed tortilla chips

Kitchen Tools:

8" x 8" baking dish

Vegetable peeler

2 1/2-quart saucepan

1-quart saucepan

Measuring cups and spoons

Instructions:

1. Preheat oven to 375 degrees F (191 degrees C). Oil baking dish and set aside.
2. Place turnips, carrots, and salt in a 2 1/2-quart saucepan. Barely cover with water and boil until tender, about 10 minutes. Drain and return to saucepan while you make the sauce.
3. In a small saucepan, heat the buttery spread or oil. Add the flour mix to the oil and stir until thickened.
4. Stirring constantly, add the rice milk, chicken broth, salt, onion powder, and dill seasoning. Cook for 1 or 2 minutes until thickened and smooth.
5. Pour sauce into the vegetable mixture and stir to combine. Spread evenly in the baking dish, and sprinkle bread crumbs or tortilla chips over vegetables.
6. Bake for 30 minutes until bubbly and slightly browned on top.

Variations:

Celery: To add celery, cut 2 stalks into 1/2" pieces, and boil with carrots and turnips. Follow the remaining directions.

Scalloped Potatoes

If you're like most people, you grew up with scalloped potatoes, and perhaps you have the perfect recipe. If not, this is a good place to start. The creamy results and the simple process make this recipe a wonderful comfort food. The outcome will be sensational and your family will love it.

Arrowroot is the thickener of choice when combined with acid forming foods such as potatoes, as cornstarch will lose its thickening ability. Experiment with additional ingredients that appeal to you. Kris

Serves: 4

Prep Time: 25 minutes

Bake Time: 1 hour 40 minutes

Ingredients:

2 lbs. potatoes, peeled and thinly sliced

---

1 large sweet onion, chopped

---

1 cup coconut milk

3/4 cup cold salt free Chicken Broth (see recipe in Mixes)

3 tablespoons grapeseed oil

3 tablespoons arrowroot starch

2 teaspoons non-salt seasoning

1 1/4 teaspoons Seasoned Salt (see recipe in Mixes)

1/4 teaspoon pepper

Kitchen Tools:

2-quart baking dish

Food processor

Vegetable peeler

2-quart saucepan

Measuring cups and spoons

Instructions:

1. Preheat oven to 350 degrees F (177 degrees C). Oil baking dish and set aside.
2. Peel potatoes and slice thinly. Use your food processor, if possible, for uniform slices.
3. Measure coconut milk, chicken broth, oil, arrowroot starch, non-salt seasoning, seasoned salt, and pepper in the saucepan. Stir to dissolve. Heat over medium heat, stirring constantly, and boil 1 minute until thickened.
4. To assemble the casserole, spread a bit of sauce in the bottom of the baking dish. Add 1/3 of the sliced potatoes, 1/3 of the chopped onion, and spread a layer of sauce. Continue layering potatoes, onions and sauce, ending with sauce spread evenly over the top.
5. Cover casserole and bake for 30 minutes. Uncover and bake for another 60 to 70 minutes, until potatoes are tender. Let stand 5 to 10 minutes before serving.

Variations:

Ham Option: Add 1 cup diced cooked ham to the layers, and follow the remaining directions.

Parsley Option: Stir 3/4 cup finely chopped fresh parsley into the sauce. Follow remaining directions.

Bacon Option: Stir 1/2 cup chopped turkey bacon into sauce. Follow remaining directions.

Cheese Option: In the last half hour of baking, sprinkle 1/2 cup of Daiya cheese of your choice on top. Follow remaining directions.

Pimento Option: Sprinkle 3 tablespoons chopped, drained pimento into the layers of potato. Sprinkle paprika on top before baking and follow remaining directions.

Red Bell Pepper & Scallion Option: Finely chop 1/2 cup red bell pepper and 1 bunch of scallions. Sprinkle into the layers of potato before baking and follow remaining directions.

Steamed Artichokes

Historians agree that artichokes originated in ancient times in Carthage, now known as Sicily or Tunisia. By 1466 artichokes could be found in Italy. From the 16th century to the end of the 20th century, the French grew artichokes and elevated them to gourmet status.

In the 16th century women were not allowed to eat this vegetable. They were reserved for men only, because it was believed artichokes were an aphrodisiac. In the 19th century, the Spanish introduced California to the artichoke and the French brought them to Louisiana. Today, all artichokes sold in the United States are grown in California.

The artichoke we eat is actually a flower bud and, if left to mature, produces a brilliant bluish-purple thistle-like bloom that is inedible. The plant itself, a perennial, can grow to a height of ten to twelve feet, but commercial plants are generally under six feet tall and four to six feet in diameter. (Thinking of a Throny Thistle? This Bud's for you!)

Fresh artichokes make a great appetizer or snack, plus they are just plain fun to eat; but if you've never had them, they can be a bit intimidating . In reality, they're easy to fix and worth the time it takes to eat them.

Look for fresh artichokes that are as blemish free as possible. You'll need a kitchen scissor to cut off the prickly ends that bite, and a steaming basket that fits into a pot with a cover. Get ready for a treat! June

Serves: 4
Prep Time: 10 minutes
Cook Time: 25 minutes

Ingredients:

4 fresh artichokes

Juice of 1 lemon
3/4 cup buttery spread

Kitchen Tools:

Kitchen scissors
Citrus juicer
Steamer basket
4 1/2-quart cooking pot

Instructions:

1. Using a kitchen scissor, clip off the tip of each sharp petal. Pull off any petals on the stem and discard. Cut the stem off, leaving about 1/2". Also, slice about 1" off the top of the artichoke.
2. Rinse each artichoke in cold water and drain.
3. Pour about 1" of water in the bottom of the cooking pot and heat to boiling. Place steamer basket in pot and position artichokes in basket. Cover and steam for 25 minutes or until petals can easily be pulled off.
4. While artichokes are steaming, melt 3 tablespoons of buttery spread in each of 4 small dipping dishes. Stir in lemon juice to taste.
5. To eat artichokes, remove outer leaves one at a time, and dip the white fleshy end in buttery mixture. Hanging onto the end of the petal, draw the petal through your front teeth, removing the soft, fleshy portion. Discard the petal and move on to the next until you get to the fuzzy base, also known as the artichoke heart.
6. When you get down to the base, scrape and discard the fuzz off the heart. Cut off any remaining stem, cut heart into bite-sized pieces, and enjoy the best part of the artichoke.

Works Cited

Thinking of a Thorny Thistle? This Bud's for You! http://www.vegparadise.com/highestperch28.html. Retrieved September 17, 2014

Summer Squash Bac-On

Coming up with new ways to use vegetables is always a challenge, particularly since we're limited in the range of vegetables we can use—either because of allergies or simply taste preferences. When we were given a beautifully perfect organic summer squash (aka yellow squash or yellow zucchini), the challenge was on. We've kept the ingredients as simple and few as possible in this dish, but the taste, texture, and presentation is definitely not ordinary. June

Serves: 4
Prep Time: 25 minutes
Bake Time: 30 minutes

Ingredients:

2 tablespoons buttery spread
4 cups yellow squash, coarsely grated
1 bunch scallions, sliced
1/2 teaspoon Seasoned Salt (see recipe in Mixes)
1/4 teaspoon pepper

---

2 slices turkey bacon, chopped

---

1 egg
2 tablespoons salt free Vegetable Broth (see recipe in Mixes)

1/4 cup gluten free bread crumbs

Kitchen Tools:

Grater or food processor

Medium skillet

Small bowl

Handheld mixer or whisk

9-cup baking dish

Instructions:

1. Preheat oven to 350 degrees F (177 degrees C). Oil baking dish and set aside.
2. Melt buttery spread in a skillet, and add the squash, scallions, seasoned salt, and pepper. Sauté on medium high heat just until soft.
3. Stir in the bacon and remove from heat. Note that turkey bacon is fully cooked so there's no need to fry it. If you are using real bacon, chop it and fry until done. Set mixture aside to cool a bit.
4. In a small bowl, beat together the egg and vegetable broth. Stir to combine and spread in the baking dish.
5. Sprinkle the bread crumbs over the top, and bake for 30 minutes or until slightly browned.

Twice Baked Potatoes

Imagine this: 22 years old, married with kids, overseas away from home, couldn't cook and Mama couldn't help, but the British nanny could. Denise introduced me to baked, stuffed potatoes complete with a lot of butter and melted cheese, and a crisp outer shell that is wonderfully edible. The secret is in peeling the potatoes and then baking them.

We swapped out rice milk for cream, buttery spread for real butter, and Daiya cheese for dairy cheese. It just doesn't get any better than this! Kris

Serves: 4

Prep Time: 10 minutes

Bake Time: 1 hour 35 minutes

Ingredients:

4 baking potatoes

1/3 cup rice milk

1/4 cup buttery spread

1 teaspoon salt

1/2 teaspoon pepper

1/4 cup Daiya Cheddar Style Shreds cheese

Kitchen Tools:

Potato peeler

Baking sheet

Measuring cups

Potato masher or handheld mixer

Medium bowl

Instructions:

1. Preheat oven to 375 degrees F (191 degrees C). Peel potatoes and place directly on center baking rack of oven. Bake for 1 hour to 1 hour 15 minutes until the potato yields to a squeeze.
2. Remove from oven and increase oven temperature to 400 degrees F (204 degrees C).
3. Using tongs or a thick clean cloth to hold the potatoes, slice potatoes lengthwise, and carefully scoop soft insides into a bowl, leaving a thin shell. Place shells on the baking sheet and set aside.
4. Add rice milk, buttery spread, salt, and pepper to bowl of cooked potato and mash until smooth. Stir in Daiya cheese.
5. Fill shells with potato mixture, and bake for 20 minutes until filling is golden brown.

Variations:

Bacon Option: Chop four slices of turkey bacon and sprinkle on top of filled shells before the final 20 minutes of baking.

Zucchini Fritters

Zucchini is a wonderfully versatile vegetable that is easy to grow and prolific in grocery stores all year around. Like other farmers in Minnesota, my mother always had a big vegetable garden, taking special pride in her weedless rows, but I wonder why she never grew or cooked zucchini. She really missed out on something special, and I think she would have liked this dish.

There are endless versions of zucchini fritter recipes available, and we've put our favorite flavor combinations together for this one. We think you'll be as delighted with the results as we are. June

Serves: 4
Prep Time: 25 minutes
Cook Time: 15 minutes

Ingredients:

2 cups grated zucchini (about 1 medium)
1/4 cup scallions, thinly sliced
3 tablespoons Daiya Mozzarella Style Shreds cheese
2 tablespoons fresh basil, minced

---

2 eggs, lightly beaten
1 tablespoon grapeseed oil

3/4 cup Bette Hagman's Featherlight Flour Mix (see recipe in Mixes)
1/4 cup quinoa flour
1 tablespoon Baking Powder (see recipe in Mixes)
1 1/2 teaspoons Seasoned Salt (see recipe in Mixes)
1/4 teaspoon black pepper

Additional grapeseed oil for cooking

Kitchen Tools:

Medium bowl

Small bowl

Measuring cups and spoons

Grater or food processor

Large griddle

Instructions:

1. Grate zucchini or use your food processor. Place zucchini in a strainer and drain well. Handful by handful, squeeze out as much moisture as possible and place in a medium bowl. Add the scallions, Daiya cheese, and fresh basil.
2. Stir in eggs and grapeseed oil.
3. In a separate small bowl, mix together the featherlight flour, quinoa flour, baking powder, seasoned salt, and black pepper. Add to the zucchini mixture and stir until thoroughly mixed. Let batter rest for 10 minutes to allow the quinoa flour to absorb moisture.
4. Coat a skillet with 1 tablespoon of grapeseed oil and heat over medium heat. Drop heaping tablespoons of batter onto hot griddle, and cook about 3 minutes until brown. Flip each fritter and cook for another 3 minutes.
5. Continue to cook batter in batches, adding additional oil to the griddle as needed. Serve warm.

Zucchini, Summer Squash & Onion Sauté

This recipe was born out of the desire to add more locally-grown vegetables into our diet in a simple, quick way that would wow our taste buds. When the Harbin Farm Stand two blocks away had their season's first zucchini and summer squash out, we decided this was the perfect time to get creative. The end result was a beautiful green and yellow side dish with loads of flavor. Kris

Serves: 6
Prep Time: 5 minutes
Cook Time: 15 minutes

Ingredients:

1 medium zucchini, quartered and sliced into 1/4" slices
1 medium summer squash, quartered and sliced into 1/4" slices
1 sweet onion, quartered and sliced
1 tablespoon grapeseed oil
2 teaspoons salt-free seasoning such as Mrs. Dash
1/2 teaspoon Seasoned Salt (see recipe in Mixes)

Kitchen Tools:

Cutting board and sharp knife
10" skillet
Measuring spoon
Spatula

Instructions:

1. Wash zucchini and summer squash with liquid soap and a soft brush to ensure all dirt and debris are removed. Quarter each the long way and slice quarters into 1/4" slices.
2. Peel onion, cut into quarters, and slice into 1/4" slices.
3. Heat oil in skillet over medium heat and add zucchini, summer squash, and onion. Sprinkle salt-free seasoning and seasoned salt over vegetables and sauté about 12 to 15 minutes, stirring often, until just tender.
4. Serve hot, garnished with fresh chopped parsley if desired.

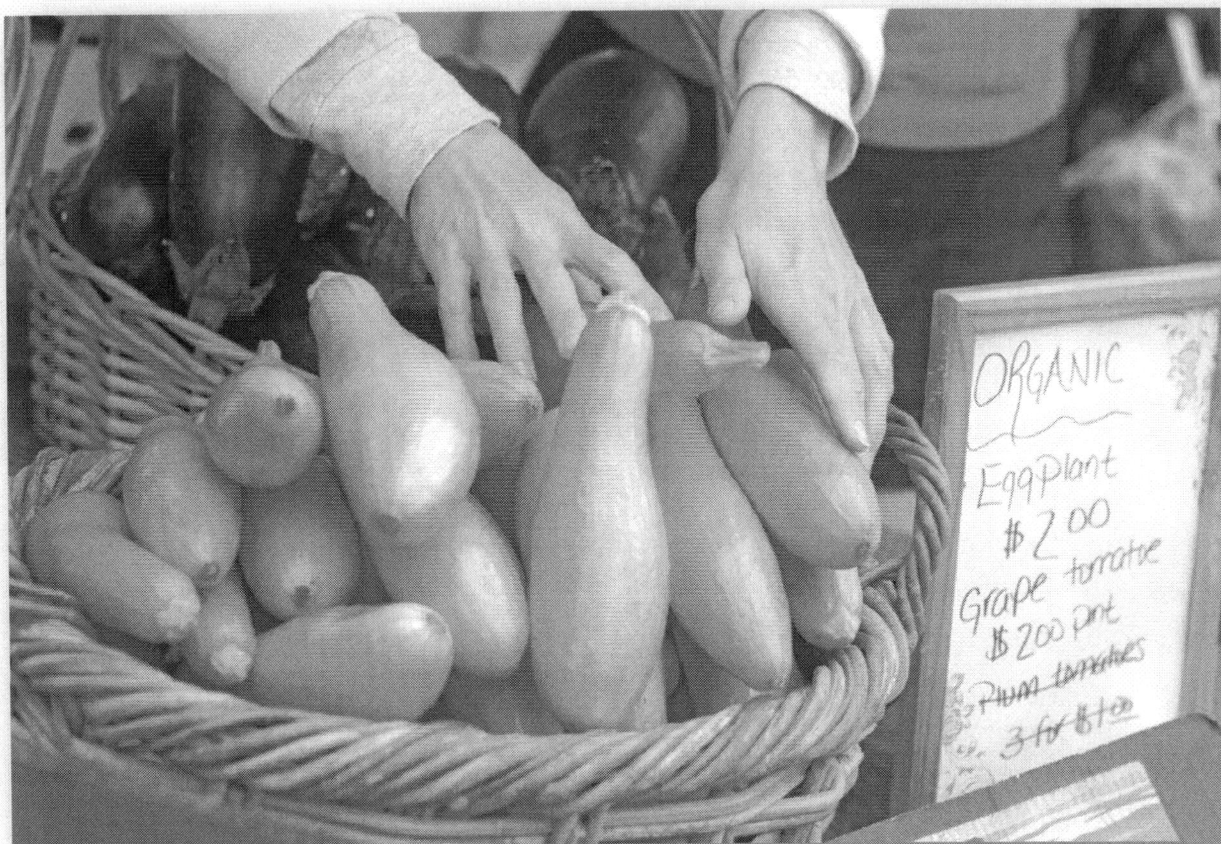
ORGANIC
Eggplant
$2.00
Grape tomatoe
$2.00 pint

Baked Asparagus With Daiya Cheese

I'll tell you right up front: once you taste asparagus fixed this way, you will never boil asparagus again. Baked with a combination of Daiya cheese and soft gluten free bread crumbs, the end result has a buttery taste and a crunchy coating.

Choose asparagus with thin stalks if possible. If not, choose asparagus with uniform sized stalks. If the stalks are slender, watch to ensure they don't burn in the baking process. June

Serves: 4

Prep Time: 10 minutes

Bake Time: 15 minutes

Ingredients:

1 lb. asparagus, washed and tough stems removed

---

1 teaspoon onion powder

1/4 teaspoon Celery Salt (see recipe in Mixes)

---

2 tablespoons Daiya Mozzarella Style Shreds cheese

2 tablespoons buttery spread

1 1/2 tablespoons soft bread crumbs

Kitchen Tools:

Nonstick baking sheet

Measuring spoons

Parchment paper (optional)

Instructions:

1. Preheat oven to 450 degrees F (232 degrees C). Lightly coat baking sheet with oil or cover with parchment paper.
2. Rinse asparagus and cut into 3" pieces. Arrange in a single layer, touching each other on the baking sheet.
3. Mix onion powder and celery salt together, and sprinkle over the asparagus. Sprinkle with Daiya cheese and bread crumbs. Dot with the buttery spread.
4. Bake uncovered until asparagus is just tender, or about 15 minutes, depending on the thickness of the asparagus. Serve warm.

Variations:

No Cheese Option: Eliminate the Daiya cheese, sprinkle with bread crumbs, and increase buttery spread to 1/4 cup.

Beautiful Veggies

There are some vegetables we don't like, a few that don't agree with us, and some we don't eat because they feed Candida. But we always celebrate when we put a new combination together in a way that is beautiful and tasty. We named this dish Beautiful because the orange, yellow, and green vegetables are in a vibrant yellow sauce. This dish goes together quickly and the flavor is stunning. Colorful side dishes with lots of flavor don't get any better than this. June

Serves: 4
Prep Time: 10 minutes
Cook Time: 12 to 15 minutes

Ingredients:
1 tablespoon buttery spread
3 carrots thinly sliced

1/2 to 1 whole yellow pepper, quartered and cut into 1/4" slices
2 tablespoons water

---

1 small zucchini halved and cut into 1/4" slices

---

1 tablespoon olive oil
1 garlic clove, minced
3/4 teaspoon salt

Kitchen Tools:

Food processor

Measuring cups and spoons

1 1/2-quart saucepan

Garlic press

Instructions:

1. Slice carrots very thin or use a food processor. Heat buttery spread in saucepan over medium heat and add carrots. Stir-fry for 5 minutes, stirring constantly.
2. Add yellow pepper and the water. Cover and continue to cook for 4 minutes, watching so it does not burn.
3. Stir in zucchini and continue to cook until veggies are almost tender. Add more water, 1 or 2 tablespoons at a time if necessary, stirring often.
4. In a separate small bowl, stir together olive oil, minced garlic, and salt. Add to vegetables and cook for 1 minute. Serve immediately.

Garlic Broccoli

This way to cook broccoli is so simple, it scarcely needs to be written down, but we all need to be reminded at times that simple can be just as good as complicated, yet takes far less time. Be sure not to overcook the broccoli. Broccoli should be a bright green and barely tender—not mushy. Kris

Serves: 4
Prep Time: 5 minutes
Cook Time: 10 to 12 minutes

Ingredients:

1 bunch fresh broccoli

---

2 tablespoons olive oil
1 or 2 large garlic cloves, minced
Salt and pepper to taste

Kitchen Tools:

4-quart saucepan
Vegetable steamer
Garlic press
Skillet

Instructions:

1. Wash broccoli and cut flowerets into serving sizes. Place in the vegetable steamer and put about an inch of water in the pan. Steam broccoli until barely tender, checking it often with your favorite fork.
2. Remove from heat and immediately rinse broccoli in cold water to stop the cooking process. Drain well.
3. Heat oil in skillet and stir-fry broccoli for a couple minutes. Add the minced garlic and stir-fry for 1 minute, stirring well to distribute garlic. Sprinkle with salt and pepper to taste and serve immediately.

Tip: Broccoli can go from "almost tender" to mushy very quickly. Broccoli will continue to cook in the vegetable steamer if over boiling water. If broccoli goes from vibrant green to dull green, broccoli is overcooked.

Mashed Parsnips, Carrots & Sweet Potatoes

We are always searching out new vegetables, and our latest discovery of parsnips proved to be a delight. Parsnips were cultivated in Roman times and come from the same biological family as carrots, parsley, and celery. Parsnips are a nutritious root vegetable, shaped like carrots but a creamy color. While parsnips are available all year around, the sweetest parsnips are those that have been in the ground until after frost.

We've combined parsnips with carrots and sweet potato for a slightly sweet, beautiful orange side dish that will complement fish, beef, pork, or chicken. June

Serves: 6

Prep Time: 10 to 15 minutes

Cook Time: 10 to 15 minutes

Ingredients:

3 medium parsnips, peeled and cut into 1/2" pieces
3 medium carrots, peeled and cut into 1/2" pieces
1 large sweet potato peeled and cut into 1/2" cubes
1 teaspoon salt

1/4 cup rice milk
1/4 cup buttery spread
1/4 teaspoon salt
1/4 teaspoon SweetLeaf English Toffee liquid stevia

Kitchen Tools:

2 1/2-quart pan
Cutting board
Your favorite chef's knife
Vegetable peeler
Measuring spoons
Potato masher

Instructions:

1. Place prepared parsnips, carrots, sweet potato, and salt in pan and barely cover with cold water. Heat to boiling, cover, and reduce heat to medium. Cook for 10 to 15 minutes or until vegetables are soft.
2. Drain vegetables and return to pan. Add rice milk, buttery spread, liquid stevia, and 1/4 teaspoon salt. Mash until smooth and serve hot.

Sautéed Zucchini With Sweet Onion & Dill

We love vegetables that don't take a lot of time to prepare and this fits the bill. It's quick and simple, appealing to the eye and delicious with a hint of dill. It's best with fresh dill, but dried dill weed will also do nicely. Kris

Serves: 4
Prep Time: 20 minutes
Cook Time: 10 to 15 minutes

Ingredients:

2 tablespoons grapeseed oil

1 1/2 cups sweet onion, chopped

3 cups zucchini cut into 1/4" slices

1/4 cup fresh dill, minced or 1 tablespoon dried dill weed

1/2 teaspoon salt

Kitchen Tools:

Sharp knife for cutting vegetables and herbs

Cutting board

Measuring cups and spoons

Medium sized skillet

Spatula (to stir and turn the vegetables)

Instructions:

1. Heat oil in a nonstick skillet on medium heat. Cook onion, stirring often for 3 minutes.
2. Add sliced zucchini and continue turning over the vegetables constantly for another 8 minutes, or until the zucchini is soft but not mushy.
3. Sprinkle salt and dill over the zucchini and stir well. Serve immediately.

Simply Asparagus

Sometimes simple is the best, and this is an uncomplicated yet delicious way to serve fresh asparagus. Choose asparagus with small stalks if possible and, if not possible, choose uniform sized stalks. Don't even consider boiling asparagus—there are much better ways to cook it and this is one of them. Be careful not to overcook it, as that "just tender" stage will enhance the gentle flavors. If you prefer a bit of tang, toss with a tablespoon of fresh lemon juice just before serving or serve with Hollandaise Sauce (see recipe in Sauces). June

Serves: 4
Prep Time: 7 minutes
Cook Time: 8 minutes

Ingredients:

1 bunch asparagus
2 tablespoons olive oil

1/2 to 3/4 teaspoon Mrs. Dash Italian Medley seasoning blend or another favorite
1/2 teaspoon sea salt

Kitchen Tools:

Small nonstick skillet
Your favorite spatula for turning the asparagus

Instructions:

1. Wash asparagus and break off any tough ends. Drain well and cut into 1 1/2" pieces.
2. Heat oil in the skillet over medium heat and add asparagus. Continue to cook, stirring often for 4 minutes, watching that it doesn't burn. Add seasonings, stir to incorporate, cover, and steam for 4 minutes until asparagus is just tender.
3. Shut off heat and serve immediately. If not serving immediately, know that the asparagus will continue to cook a bit even with the heat off.

Variations:

Lemon Option: Just before serving, toss with a tablespoon of fresh lemon juice.

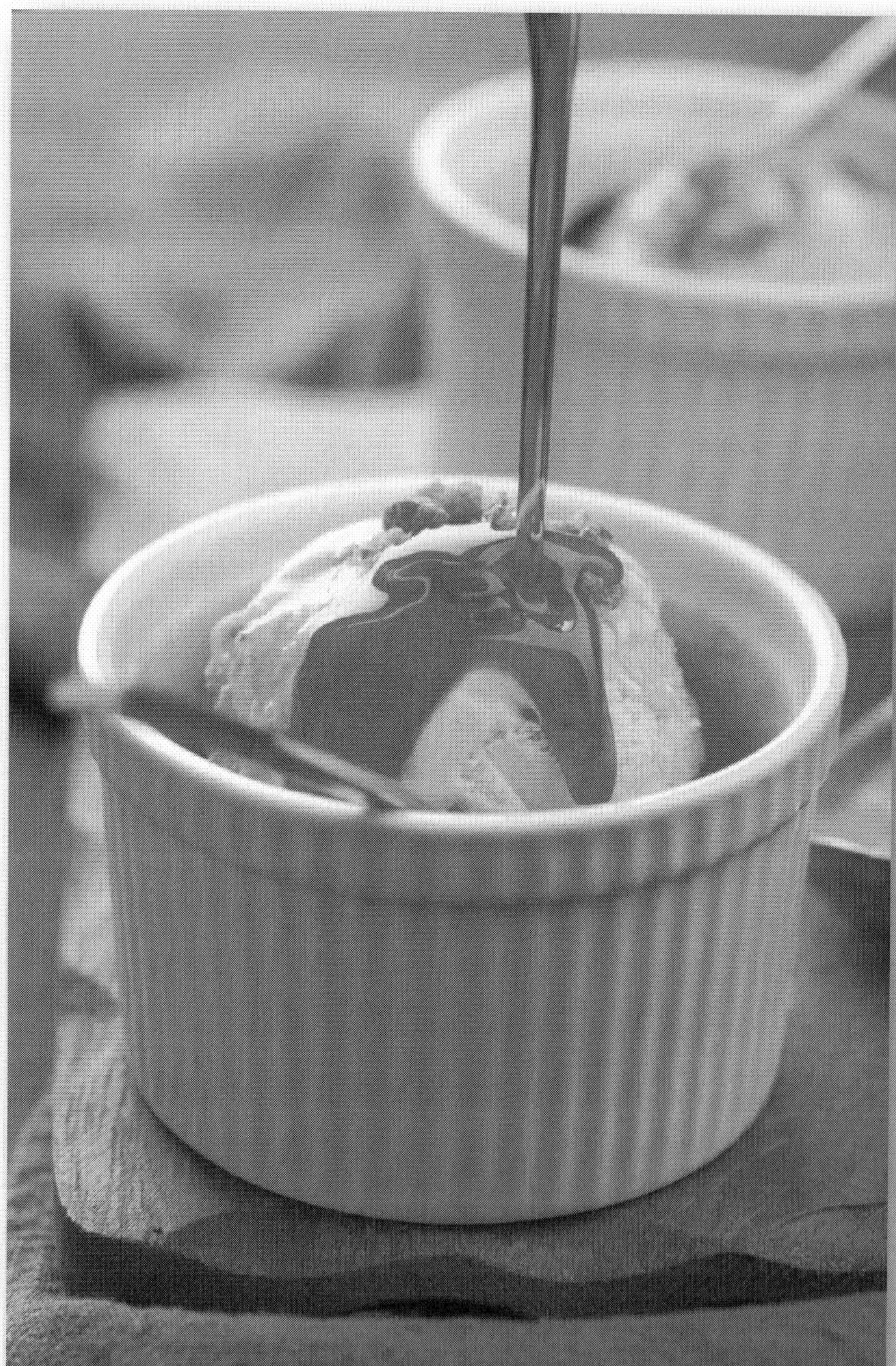

SAUCES

Sauces can be either sweet or savory, and a good sauce will turn even the most simple and unadorned food into something elegant and special. A carefully chosen sauce will offer a contrasting taste or texture to a main dish, vegetable, or dessert. The esthetic factor should not be discounted either, as it's been proven that food with eye appeal tastes better than unattractive or boring food.

In this section, you will find sweet sauces to use on pancakes, as frosting or between layers of desserts. Let your imagination go wild and layer sauces for a new taste.

Savory sauces include creamed sauces, dressings for your salad, sauces designed to be baked into main course dishes, and even a white pizza sauce. We are confident you'll go to this section often to give even mundane foods a tantalizing boost.

Sweet Berry Sauce

This recipe was born out of a need to give us more space in our freezer. It was an early Saturday morning, and we had not had Belgian Waffles for quite some time. Kris is sensitive to all sugars, and as she explained, waffles without a sweet syrup or topping is like wearing a tuxedo without a tie, or going to the ball without wearing your makeup.

I was feeling creative, and a bag of frozen mixed berries presented an opportunity to invent a sweet tasting sauce that had a low glycemic index. Until this point, coconut syrup was her only choice to top waffles or pancakes, and it was a treat to have something different. With her first taste, she smiled broadly and declared, "A dollop of cold coconut cream on top, and I'd think I was at IHOP!" An endorsement doesn't get any better than that! June

Makes: 2 1/2 cups
Prep Time: 10 minutes
Cook Time: 5 minutes

Ingredients:

4 cups frozen mixed berries, thawed and drained

1/2 cup berry juice drained from thawed berries

1/4 cup water
1 tablespoon plus 1 teaspoon cornstarch
1 tablespoon vegetable glycerine
1 tablespoon coconut nectar
1/2 teaspoon blueberry juice concentrate
1 1/4 teaspoons SweetLeaf Lemon Drop stevia

Kitchen Tools:

1-quart saucepan

Measuring cups and spoons

Your favorite stirring spoon

Instructions:

1. Thaw and drain the berries, retaining the juice. Set the berries aside.
2. In the saucepan, combine the berry juice, water, cornstarch, vegetable glycerine, coconut nectar, blueberry juice concentrate, and liquid stevia until cornstarch is dissolved.
3. Heat over medium heat, stirring constantly and boil 1 minute. Add the berries and heat through.
4. Serve warm over Belgian waffles, pancakes, or ice cream. Or make a double batch, chill, and use as a filling between cake layers or jellyroll.

Caramel Syrup

This syrup is so easy to make with just two ingredients, but the effect is high impact. Use it over ice cream or muffins that need a bit of sweetness, or drizzle over cake or frosting.

Tapioca syrup needs to be refrigerated after opening, so allow it to come to room temperature when you're working with it. Don't try to cut time by microwaving it, however. It will totally change the consistency! Kris

Makes: 1/4 cup
Prep Time: 5 minutes

Ingredients:

1/4 cup tapioca syrup
3/4 teaspoon SweetLeaf English Toffee liquid stevia

Kitchen Tools:

Small bowl
Measuring cup and spoon

Instructions:

1. Stir the tapioca syrup and liquid stevia until well combined. Store any leftover syrup in the refrigerator. Let come to room temperature to work with it—don't microwave or the tapioca syrup will turn into a stiffened mass.
2. Serve over ice cream, muffins, hot cereal, pancakes, or waffles—whatever needs a bit of sweetness.

Choco-Coco-Berry Frosting

When we went looking for a frosting recipe that was sugar free, dairy free, and didn't call for cream cheese or sugar-free pudding mix, we came up empty handed. With all the knowledge out there, I wouldn't have imagined we'd have to figure this out without any pre-established guidelines. There are times when I wish I had the knowledge of food chemistry under my belt, as without it, any creation is a matter of trial and error.

For this recipe, we put together ingredients for sweetness, stability, texture, and spreadability with some sweet results. The chocolate, coconut, and chocolate raspberry stevia make it perfect to spread on any muffin or cookie that needs a bit of chocolate contrast and sweetness. June

Makes: 1 cup
Prep Time: 10 minutes

Ingredients:

1/2 cup plus 1 tablespoon unsweetened coconut flakes
1/4 cup plus 2 tablespoons cocoa powder
1/4 cup plus 2 tablespoons tapioca syrup
1/4 cup plus 2 tablespoons buttery spread
1 tablespoon Frontier Non-Alcoholic Vanilla
1/2 teaspoon plus 4 drops SweetLeaf Chocolate Raspberry liquid stevia
1/8 teaspoon salt

Kitchen Tools:

Small bowl
Measuring cups and spoons

Instructions:

1. In a small bowl, vigorously stir all ingredients to combine. Spread on cookies or muffins, and store anything frosted covered, in a single layer.

Lemon Cake Filling

This filling was adapted from a recipe in Betty Crocker's New Picture Cookbook, published by McGraw Hill Book Company, circa 1961. Betty certainly knew her stuff and taught many young women not only how to cook, but also how to entertain and still look nice for her husband when he came home from work. June Cleaver in her daytime pearls, probably took her cue from Betty. Times have so changed, but the recipes still endure, and with some changes to the original recipe, the fresh lemony flavor makes a great filling between layers of cake. You'll also find this recipe as the filling for our Jellyroll. Kris

Makes: 2 cups
Prep Time: 30 minutes
Cook Time: 25 minutes
Cooling Time: 30 minutes

Ingredients:

2 tablespoons grated lemon zest
3 tablespoons fresh lemon juice

---

1 1/2 cups water
3 tablespoons vegetable glycerine
1/4 cup cornstarch
1 1/8 teaspoons SweetLeaf liquid stevia
1/2 teaspoon SweetLeaf Lemon Drop liquid stevia

---

2 egg yolks, slightly beaten

---

1 tablespoon Frontier Non-Alcoholic Vanilla

Kitchen Tools:

Whisk or handheld mixer

Measuring cups and spoons

Grater for lemon zest

Citrus juicer

1 1/2-quart saucepan

Instructions:

1. Wash and rinse the lemon. Using a fairly fine side of the grater, make the lemon zest. Measure out 2 tablespoons and set aside. Juice the lemon, measure out 3 tablespoons, and set aside.
2. Stir the water, vegetable glycerine, cornstarch, and liquid stevias in the saucepan until the cornstarch is dissolved. Cook over medium heat, stirring constantly, until mixture thickens. Boil 1 minute.
3. In a bowl, whisk egg yolks until broken down. While whisking vigorously, pour at least half the hot mixture into the egg yolks. Return all to the saucepan and reducing heat a bit, boil for 1 minute longer, stirring constantly.
4. Remove from heat and stir in the lemon zest, lemon juice, and vanilla. Let cool, stirring occasionally as it thickens, and use as filling between cake layers or jellyroll.

Chocolate Coconut Cream Frosting

Sugar is the perfect base for traditional frostings because it provides not only sweetness, but also substantial mass that can be manipulated through heating or with the addition of other ingredients. It required a lot of thinking to figure out a combination of ingredients that would give us a sweet, satisfying frosting, and yet keep within our list of permitted foods.

If you've never had coconut cream, you're in for a treat. It can be found in the canned section of most grocery stores and in all oriental stores. When coconut cream is chilled for 24 hours, the "cream" comes to the top and becomes the thick base for this frosting, which is very easy to make, light and tasty, but also deceptively rich.

It does have some limitations. It will lose its integrity at room temperature, so it must be kept refrigerated and is best used as needed, just as you would treat whipped cream. You can frost a cake with it, and put it between layers, but you will need to eat it within 3 days. We think you'll like its creamy texture and sweetness, which tops off a cake or muffins beautifully. June

Makes: 4 cups
Prep Time: 10 minutes

Ingredients:
1 14-oz. can well chilled coconut cream (at least 20 g. fat per 1/2 cup) (resist the urge to shake it)
1/4 cup cocoa powder
1 teaspoon SweetLeaf English Toffee liquid stevia
3 tablespoons Frontier Non-Alcoholic Vanilla
Pinch of salt

Kitchen Tools:
Medium bowl
Measuring cups and spoons
Handheld mixer

Instructions:

1. Chill coconut cream in the refrigerator for at least 24 hours, to allow the cream to rise to the top and the liquid to sink. Remove from refrigerator and open without shaking or stirring. Scoop the congealed coconut cream into a medium bowl, but reserve the liquid.
2. Add the cocoa powder, stevia, vanilla, and salt to the coconut cream. Stir well until smooth and, if too thick, add a tablespoon of leftover coconut liquid until the right consistency is achieved. Keep chilled until you are ready to serve.

Hollandaise Sauce

Hollandaise Sauce is so easy to make and adds a very special element to a dish, but requires some care when making. Use well-chilled or even frozen buttery spread, stir constantly, and use only very low heat. It only takes a few minutes to make hollandaise, but it cannot be rushed.

This sauce is the perfect accent for cooked greens of any kind, turning same-old into something elegant. Experiment with thin toasted gluten-free bread, topped with Canadian bacon, cooked spinach with lemon pepper, a soft-fried egg and hollandaise. June

Serves: 4

Prep Time: 10 minutes

Ingredients:

2 egg yolks

3 tablespoons fresh lemon juice

1/4 teaspoon salt

1/4 teaspoon onion powder

1/2 cup very cold or frozen buttery spread

Kitchen Tools:

Small saucepan

Measuring spoons and cups

Citrus juicer

Whisk

Instructions:

1. Put egg yolks, lemon juice, salt, and onion powder in a small saucepan. Whisk to break down egg yolks and mix well.
2. Add half the cold buttery spread and turn the heat on low (seriously, don't try to rush this process by turning up the heat). Whisking constantly, heat gently to melt the butter and give the egg yolks time to cook and thicken the sauce.
3. Add the remainder of the cold buttery spread and continue whisking until buttery spread is melted and sauce is thick. If you've followed the directions to this point, the buttery spread is properly melted, and the sauce is not thick, turn up the heat just a tad to cook egg yolks. Whisk constantly until sauce is thick. Remove from heat.

Note: If sauce separates, slowly stir in 1 teaspoon water while heating on low. Store any leftover hollandaise in the refrigerator. To reuse, stir a tablespoon of boiling water into leftover hollandaise and serve. Do not microwave sauce.

Variations:

Dill Option: Add 2 tablespoons fresh minced dill to finished sauce.

Alfredo Sauce

This is probably the best Alfredo Sauce I've ever had—far better than any packaged mix! This sauce is smooth and creamy, kissed with garlic and fresh parsley. It is wonderfully neutral, so you can add your own herbs and veggies to jazz it up!

We came up with this recipe one night when I was desperate for a pasta meal, and Alfredo was sounding really good. I looked at the back of an Alfredo package mix we had forgotten to throw out and converted an old recipe from Betty Crocker's New Picture Cookbook, published by McGraw Hill Book Company, circa 1961. Have fun with it and make it your own by adding your favorite herbs or other seasonings! Kris

Serves: 4
Prep Time: 10 minutes
Cook Time: 15 minutes

Ingredients:

1/2 onion, chopped
2 tablespoons oil

---

3 garlic cloves, minced
1 cup salt free Chicken Broth (see recipe in Mixes)

---

1 egg
1/2 cup coconut milk

---

1 cup rice milk
2 tablespoons cornstarch

---

2 cups Daiya Mozzarella Style Shreds cheese

1/2 teaspoon salt
Pepper to taste
3 tablespoons fresh parsley, chopped

Kitchen Tools:

1-quart saucepan

Measuring cups and spoons

Garlic press

Whisk or handheld mixer

Instructions:

1. Heat oil over medium heat and sauté onion until soft and translucent.
2. Turn up heat to medium or medium high, and stir in chicken broth and garlic.
3. In a small bowl, beat egg, and combine with coconut milk. Stir into onion mixture.
4. Dissolve cornstarch in rice milk in a cup, and stir into onion mixture. Stirring constantly, bring to a gentle rolling boil, and cook for 3 to 5 minutes until it is the consistency of thin pudding.
5. Add Daiya cheese and stir until melted.
6. Add salt and pepper to taste, and stir in the fresh, chopped parsley.
7. Serve hot over your favorite cooked gluten-free pasta.

Variations:

Chicken and Pasta: Serve grilled chicken over gluten-free pasta, and top with Alfredo Sauce.

Broccoli Ala Alfredo: Serve Alfredo Sauce over hot cooked broccoli and gluten-free pasta.

Mixed Vegetables & Pasta: Sauté your favorite combination of mixed vegetables and stir into Alfredo Sauce. Serve over gluten-free pasta.

Tip: When choosing garlic, look for cloves that are firm to the touch. Look at the bottom of the clump and press your thumb into any that appear to be dark under the white skin. If it yields to your thumb, choose another garlic.

Tip: To easily peel garlic, separate the cloves and flatten with the broad side of a large knife. The peeling will come off easily. Cut off the hard nubby end of the blunt end of the clove. Save the peelings and discarded ends in a closable freezer bag for vegetable, chicken, or beef broth.

Crepe Cream Sauce

Early in our journey into healthy, gluten free, dairy-free foods, we determined not to have to give up all the foods we really loved. Since a good cream sauce is so versatile, we put both our brains together to develop the very best taste and smoothest texture possible. We combined chicken broth with the creaminess of coconut milk, thickened it with cornstarch, and added onions and seasonings for an end product that lends itself to complimenting vegetables or our Chicken Crepes recipe. Don't omit the fresh chopped parsley, as it brings all the flavors together beautifully. Use it as a base for your own creative creamed dishes. Kris

Serves: 4
Prep Time: 10 minutes
Cook Time: 15 minutes

Ingredients:

1/2 onion, finely chopped
2 tablespoons oil

---

1 1/2 cups salt free Chicken Broth (see recipe in Mixes)

---

1 egg
1/2 cup coconut milk
1/2 cup salt free Chicken Broth
1/4 cup cornstarch

---

3 tablespoons fresh chopped parsley
1 teaspoon salt
1/2 teaspoon pepper

Kitchen Tools:

2 1/2-quart saucepan

Measuring cups and spoons

Whisk or handheld mixer

Small bowl

Instructions:

1. In the saucepan, heat oil over medium or medium low heat. Add onions, and stirring often, sauté about 5 minutes until onions are soft and translucent.
2. Turn up heat to medium or medium high, and stir in 1 1/2 cups chicken broth.
3. In a small bowl, beat egg and combine with coconut milk, 1/2 cup cold chicken broth and cornstarch. Stir into onion mixture and combine well.
4. Bring to a gentle rolling boil, reduce heat, and stirring occasionally, cook on low for 2 minutes until it is the consistency of thin pudding.
5. Stir in chopped parsley, salt and pepper.
6. Serve as part of the recipe for Chicken Crepes With Mixed Vegetables & Parsley (see recipe in Chicken section) or over your favorite cooked vegetable, garnished with chopped parsley.

Variations:

Dill Cream Sauce: Substitute fresh chopped dill or 1 tablespoon dried dill weed for the parsley and serve over cooked broccoli.

Herbed Salad Dressing

When I realized the extent of the foods I could no longer have, the one thing I missed the most was my beloved Ranch Dressing. Commercial dressings are out, as all of them have ingredients I can't have, and the primary offender is vinegar. After having a few hissy fits where nobody could see me, I discovered apricot kernel oil and fresh lemon juice squeezed on my salad was satisfying, although definitely nothing like Ranch Dressing.

In an effort to give me more choices, my mom put this dressing together. It has no vinegar or lemon juice, but is tasty and offers a quick-to-make alternative. It is a thick, very green dressing, and is equally wonderful on cooked chicken or turkey burgers. As always, make it your own with your favorite herbs. For a bold flavor, use fresh herbs instead of dried. Kris

Makes: 1/3 cup

Prep Time: 5 minutes

Ingredients:

1/3 cup apricot kernel oil

2 tablespoons fresh parsley, chopped

2 teaspoons dried dill weed

1 teaspoon onion powder

3/4 teaspoon dried oregano

1/2 teaspoon sea salt

1/8 teaspoon ground pepper

Kitchen Tools:

Small bowl

Measuring cup and spoons

Small whisk

Instructions:

1. Measure all ingredients into the bowl and whisk vigorously. Store leftovers tightly covered in the refrigerator. Stir before using. Drizzle over salad greens, avocado, burgers, cooked chicken, or broiled steak.

Variations:

More Tang: For a more tangy dressing, add 2 tablespoons fresh squeezed lemon juice.

Lemon Oil Salad Dressing

Delicious salad dressings need not have mysterious ingredients to be satisfying. This recipe calls for fresh squeezed lemon juice, your favorite oil, and simple spices, but the results are really taste bud popping. Don't try to cut corners with bottled lemon juice—part of the delight of this dressing is the fresh taste, and you can't get that out of a bottle.

This recipe can be a finished product or a launch pad for your own dressing. Be creative and make it your own with your favorite fresh chopped herbs or other flavor combinations that please your palate. June

Makes: 1/2 cup

Prep Time: 5 minutes

Ingredients:

1/4 cup fresh squeezed lemon juice

1/4 cup of your favorite oil

1 teaspoon non-salt garlic & herb seasoning such as Mrs. Dash

1/2 teaspoon Seasoned Salt (see recipe in Mixes)

1/4 teaspoon onion powder

1/8 teaspoon ground pepper

Kitchen Tools:

Small bowl

Measuring cup and spoons

Small whisk

Instructions:

1. Measure all ingredients into a bowl and whisk vigorously. Store leftovers tightly covered in the refrigerator. Stir before using, and use within a couple of days.

Margarine

Finding a buttery spread that didn't have soy, dairy, or other forbidden ingredients was a frustrating struggle. Kris had one brand available to her, but it was pretty expensive to bake with. We were thrilled to see a recipe for Homemade Margarine in a Living Without's Gluten Free & More magazine, and deeply grateful to J'Marinde Shephard who laboriously designed this allergy-friendly margarine. We made a few changes to suit our taste, and added xanthan gum, which we feel improves the texture. The down side to xanthan gum is that it discourages the margarine from melting like butter.

This recipe calls for liquid lecithin, which functions as an emulsifier, thickener, and stabilizer. Soy lecithin is most commonly found, but if you search the internet, you will find sunflower lecithin, which is what we have used.

We especially like the flavor of this margarine for cooking and baking, and keep it on hand in the freezer. Our thanks to Ms. Shephard for sharing her recipe with the world, and graciously giving us permission to include it in our book. June

Makes: 1 1/2 cups

Prep Time: 15 minutes

Freezer Time: 2 hours

Ingredients:

1/2 cup olive oil
1/2 cup coconut milk
1/4 cup sunflower oil
1/4 cup grapeseed oil
1 tablespoon coconut oil, melted
1 teaspoon sunflower liquid lecithin
1 teaspoon xanthan gum
1/2 teaspoon salt (or less to taste)
Dash ground turmeric (less than 1/8 teaspoon)

Kitchen Tools:

Blender
Measuring cups and spoons

Instructions:

1. Combine all ingredients in a blender, and blend on medium high for at least 2 minutes until well blended and creamy. Immediately pour into a shallow container, close tightly, and freeze. Store margarine in the freezer.
2. To make "buttery spread curls," draw a butter curler knife across the top of the frozen margarine.

Pesto Sauce

Pesto sauce is actually a paste and is incredibly easy to make. It can be frozen for later use if you prefer. It's best to make when basil is in season in late summer (you can get a big bunch of it for little cost), but some quantities of fresh basil are available year around. Don't try to substitute dried basil for fresh—it simply won't work.

Pesto's vivid green color and smooth garlic taste make it a natural to combine with cooked, drained, hot pasta. It's also great on chicken breasts, fish, as a pizza sauce, or any dish that needs a bit of zip. Make up a batch and then experiment to make your own favorite pesto dishes. June

Makes: 1 cup

Prep Time: 30 minutes

Ingredients:

3 cups packed fresh basil leaves

3/4 cup packed fresh parsley

1/2 cup Daiya Mozzarella Style Shreds cheese

1/2 cup pine nuts

1/4 cup olive oil

1/4 cup melted buttery spread

3/4 teaspoons salt

2 to 6 large cloves fresh garlic (depending on taste)

Kitchen Tools:

Food processor or blender

Measuring cups

Instructions:

1. Wash the basil and parsley, and remove the leaves from the stems. Drain or pat dry with paper towels.
2. Combine all ingredients in a food processor or blender, arranging ingredients to give the blade optimum efficiency. Process on whatever speed works best for about 2 minutes, scraping down bowl as needed, until you have a smooth paste.
3. Refrigerate or freeze any leftover pesto. When ready to use, spoon the quantity you will need into a bowl and add a tablespoon of very hot water, stirring to melt sauce. Toss with hot pasta, vegetables, or top fish or chicken. It also makes a great pizza sauce.

Note: If you're short on basil leaves, replace up to 1 cup of basil with 1 cup fresh parsley.

White Pizza Sauce

I love pizza! But after learning I couldn't eat tomatoes along with so many of my other favorite foods, I was determined not to miss out on all of life's simple pleasures. I had never had white pizza before, and, in desperation, I flipped through a dozen cookbooks looking for something I could use as a sauce. In the end, I simply began putting together ingredients until I reached the consistency and taste I wanted. This sauce is infused with the wonderful flavors of onion and garlic, and is the consistency of a velvety cottage cheese. My mother loves this sauce and has put it on top of tomato-based pizza sauce to create a flavorful "pink" sauce! Kris

Makes: Enough for a small pizza

Prep Time: 5 minutes

Cook Time: 10 minutes

Ingredients:

2 tablespoons oil

2 tablespoons finely diced onion

---

1 tablespoon plus 1 1/2 teaspoons any gluten free flour mix

1/4 teaspoon Seasoned Salt (see recipe in Mixes)

1/8 teaspoon pepper

1/2 cup rice milk

1 small garlic clove, minced or 1/2 teaspoon garlic powder

Kitchen Tools:

Small saucepan

Cutting board and sharp knife

Garlic press

Instructions:

1. Heat oil in small saucepan, add diced onion, and sauté until soft and translucent, stirring often.
2. Mix flour, salt, and pepper together, and stir into onion and oil mixture. Stir until smooth.
3. Gradually add rice milk, stirring constantly until thick.
4. Add garlic and continue stirring for 1 minute.
5. Remove from heat and let sit for a minute to thicken. Spread on your favorite pizza crust, add toppings, and bake as desired.

Red Bell Pepper Sauce

A good sauce can transform an ordinary dish into a gourmet food, and this sauce is the perfect accompaniment for meatloaf, hamburgers, or any cut of beef. The pine nuts give it a stable base, bell peppers and red onion make it a beautiful orange color, lime juice offers just the right amount of tang, and the beef broth and stevia knit all the flavors together.

When red bell peppers are on sale, we stock up and make a large batch of this sauce, which freezes well until we need it. This sauce takes a bit of time to make, but it is so worth the effort. June

Makes: 1 1/2 cups
Broiling and Processing Time: Approximately 45 minutes
Cooling Time: 20 minutes
Peeling Time: 10 minutes

Ingredients:

2 large red bell peppers (square with 4 equal sides for ease in broiling)

---

1 large red onion, chopped
1 1/2 teaspoons oil

---

3 garlic cloves, minced

1/4 cup pine nuts
2 tablespoons fresh lime juice
1 1/2 teaspoons Seasoned Salt (see recipe in Mixes)
1/8 teaspoon cayenne pepper (optional)
5 drops SweetLeaf Apricot Nectar liquid stevia

1/3 cup salt free Beef Broth (see recipe in Mixes)

Kitchen Tools:

Food processor

Broiler pan

Sturdy brown paper bag

Measuring cups and spoons

Small skillet

Small saucepan

Instructions:

1. Turn on your oven's broiler.
2. To prepare red peppers, wash them, and place them whole on the broiler pan. Broil each side of the pepper close to heat until each side is blistered and blackened, which makes the peppers easy to peel. Watch them closely and turn each pepper with tongs. Total broiling time will be about 45 minutes.
3. While peppers are broiling or resting, chop the red onion and sauté in a small skillet with the oil until soft. Add the garlic and continue to cook for 1 minute more. Transfer to a food processor.
4. Add the pine nuts, lime juice, seasoned salt, cayenne pepper, and liquid stevia. Process on high for 2 minutes until smooth, scraping down sides as needed. Add the beef broth and process briefly.
5. Remove peppers from the oven and transfer to a brown paper bag. Roll the bag shut and leave the peppers to "sweat" and cool off, at least 20 minutes. This step allows the blackened skin to come away from the meat of the peppers, making the peeling process easier.
6. When peppers are cooled, peel the blackened skin off the peppers and discard. Peeling is a bit tedious, but is made easier if you peel under a slow stream of cold water. Discard the seeds, rinse off peppers and drain well. You should have about 1 1/4 cups of peppers. Put in your food processor with the other ingredients, and process on high for 1 minute.
7. Transfer mixture to a small saucepan and heat. Serve over meatloaf, hamburgers, fish, or in any dish you would normally use a tomato base.

Tip: Because this is a fairly labor intensive dish but deliciously versatile, make a double batch and freeze what you can't use immediately. It freezes well in ice cube trays for individual serving sizes. Once frozen, transfer to an airtight container.

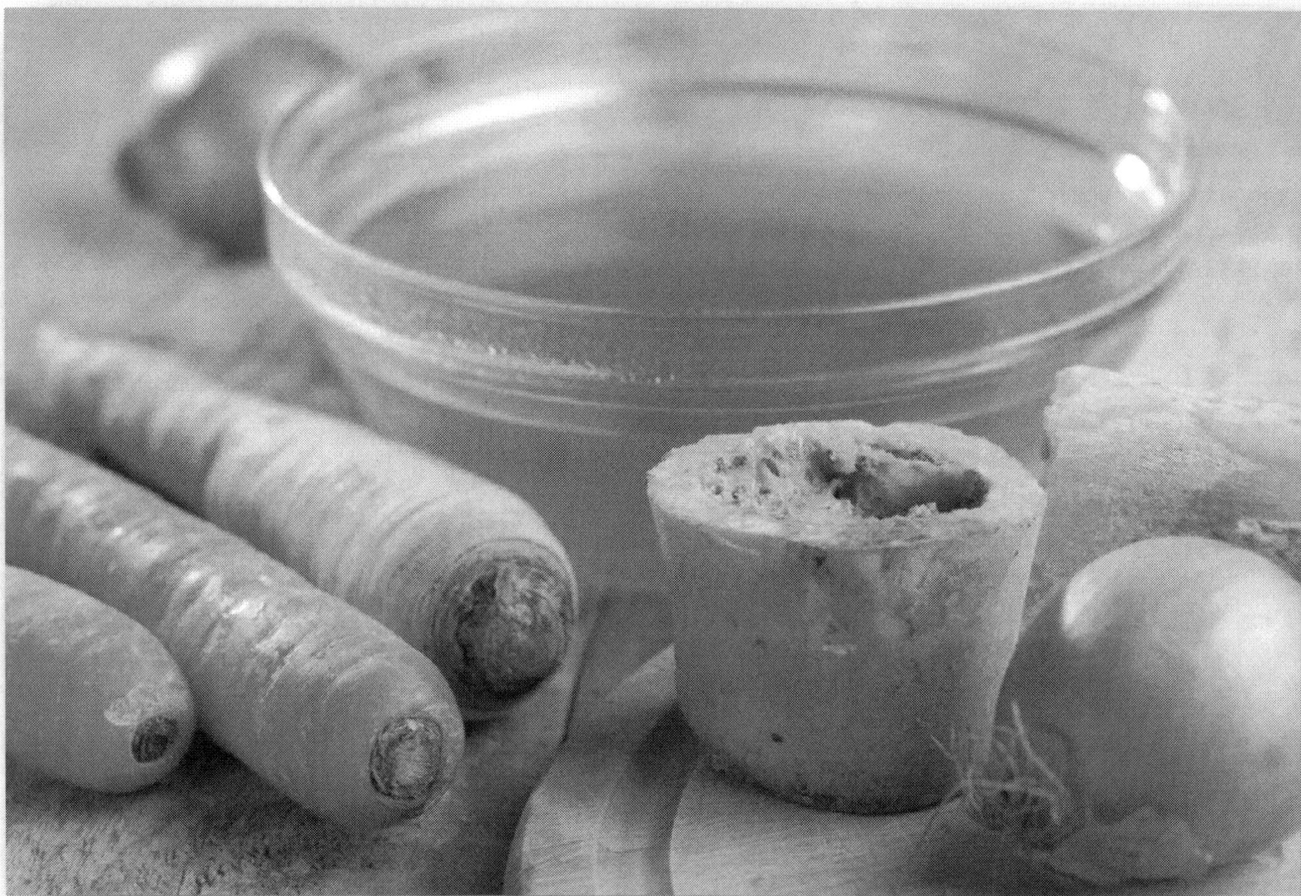

MIXES

Between the pages of this section are recipes for the chicken, beef, and vegetable broth that form the base for many of our savory dishes and sauces. Also included are the three flour mixes we use the most, as well as spice and herb combinations.

You'll find salt mixtures that enhance your dishes, herb combinations, spices, and a simple recipe for baking powder. With the exception of the broths, all these mixes go together in less than 10 minutes, and can be stored in a cupboard for months.

Beef Broth

If you have ever read the label of conventional beef broths, you were probably as annoyed as we were with the unnecessary and downright harmful ingredients. Here's a sample of one of the leading brand's Beef Broth: Salt, Monosodium Glutamate, Hydrolyzed Soy Protein, Hydrolyzed Whey Protein (Milk) and Wheat Bran Protein, Hydrolyzed Wheat Protein, Hydrolyzed Corn Protein, Dextrose, Onion Powder, Autolyzed Yeast Extract, Caramel Color, Natural Flavor (this can be anything), Partially Hydrogenated Soybean Oil, Thiamine Hydrochloride, Disodium Inosinate, Disodium Guanylate. My motto is, "If I can't pronounce it, I don't want to eat it." That is precisely why we take the extra time to make our own broth. Plus, we love the flavor and convenience of pulling what we need out of the freezer.

We save all our vegetable scraps and peelings in gallon sized resealable plastic bags in the freezer. The rules for what to save and what should be in the garbage disposal involve common sense. You can use wilted vegetables, as long as they are not obviously rotten, dirty, or contaminated. Wash all vegetables before peeling or slicing. Keep the "sweet" vegetables in equal or higher proportion to "strong tasting" vegetables. For example, carrots, celery, apple cores and peelings, sweet peppers, winter squash, and onions will give your broth a gentle sweetness. On the other hand, too much cabbage, broccoli, or strong greens will give your broth an unpleasant overtone.

We look for inexpensive beef cuts on sale and then buy in quantity, freezing it for future use if we're not ready to make broth immediately. My last great find was at one of those large warehouse stores when stew meat was less than half the cost of ground beef.

You'll find some guidelines below. June

Prep Time: 1 to 2 hours (including straining at the end)
Cook Time: 4 hours or longer

Ingredients:

6 quarts of liquid from list below

Approximately 10 lbs. beef meat (stew meat works best)

2 to 4 1-gallon freezer bags of saved vegetable scraps

4 to 6 bay leaves

Kitchen Tools:

Large stockpot

Large strainer

Splatter screen

Large bowl or stockpot to drain broth into

Several freezer containers in sizes that makes sense for you

Potato masher

Instructions:

1. Thaw any liquids you have been saving and heat in stockpot.
2. Thaw beef if necessary and cut into 2" to 3" pieces. Thaw vegetable scraps in the microwave and add to the stockpot along with the bay leaves. Liquid should almost cover the beef and vegetables, as additional juices will be naturally generated upon cooking. **Do not add salt.**
3. Turn stove on high until mixture boils, cover, and reduce heat to low to allow beef and vegetables to simmer for no less than 4 hours, and up to 6 hours to make a richer broth. There's no exact science here—just make sure the liquid doesn't boil away. Remove from heat and let cool a bit.
4. Place a sturdy strainer over a large, deep bowl or pan. Ladle cooked vegetables and liquid into the strainer a few cups at a time. Press down to squeeze out juices (a potato masher works great here), and when well drained, dispose of the pulp and meat. Repeat the process until the entire batch has been strained.
5. Wash out the original stockpot or use another large pot or bowl. Using a splatter screen, strain the liquid a second time into the pot to eliminate seeds and any small particles. If your freezer space is at a premium, return the broth to the stove and continue to cook until the broth is reduced by half. This intensifies the flavor and, upon use, simply use 1 part broth with 1 part water.
6. Cool broth in the freezer long enough for the fat to form a solid layer on the top and remove the fat. Or if you are out of time and/or patience, simply pour broth into freezer containers and freeze. Fat will come to the top. To easily remove fat, microwave frozen broth on high for 1 to 2 minutes and "peel" off the fat.
7. Label each container with not only what it is, but also the date to make it easier to rotate broth. Also note on the label if you've reduced the broth so it is extra rich. Use in soups, gravies, casseroles, and in place of water in most savory recipes.

Usable Ingredients:

Carrot peelings and ends

Celery tops and leaves

Onion skins (no dirt please)

Garlic skins and ends

Sweet pepper ends and insides

Turnip peelings

Zucchini ends

Swiss chard ends

Asparagus ends

Shallot peelings

Summer squash ends

Cucumber seeds and ends

Apple, peach or pear peelings and cores

Seeds and the stringy pulp from the center of winter squash

Stems from fresh herbs such as parsley, dill, basil, sage and thyme

Cooked vegetables that won't get eaten within a couple days

Less than perfect outer lettuce leaves

Liquids to Use:

Liquid from canned vegetables

Water from cooked fresh vegetables

Filtered water

Ingredients to Limit:

Broccoli stalks cut into 1" pieces (strong flavor)

Cabbage leaves (strong flavor)

Water potatoes are cooked in (starchy and turns broth dark)

What Not to Include:

Banana peelings

Cucumber peelings

Citrus peels

Tough stems from winter squash

Avocado shells

Potato peelings (starchy and turns broth dark)

Baking Powder

Before becoming aware of gluten issues, I would have never thought to check baking powder for gluten. Baking powder is a combination of baking soda, cream of tartar, and a starch, which can be cornstarch, potato starch, or wheat starch. Additionally, some brands contain aluminum. In the past 20 years, there has been a great deal of research into the dangers of aluminum toxicity, and high levels of aluminum have been found in the brains of Alzheimer and Parkinson's patients. That was enough to send me looking for a safer alternative.

We particularly like this Baking Powder recipe because the starch is arrowroot starch, but you could substitute cornstarch if you prefer. We choose to limit our corn intake as much as possible since it causes reactions in Kris in whole form, and experience has showed us that consistently consuming a food often leads to an allergy to that product. If you prefer to purchase baking powder, do your research and choose brands that are without harmful ingredients. June

Prep Time: 5 minutes

Ingredients:

2 parts cream of tartar

2 parts arrowroot starch (aka arrowroot powder or arrowroot flour)

1 part baking soda

Kitchen Tools:

Measuring spoons

Convenient container to store it in

Instructions:

1. Measure out ingredients and mix thoroughly. Store in an airtight, labeled container.

Chicken Broth

We have yet to understand why commercial broths need to have sugar and yeast in them, or worse yet, MSG. Chicken broth is easy to make, but requires a bit of dedicated time, so plan to start this process first thing in the morning rather than after your evening meal.

We save all our vegetable scraps and peelings in gallon sized resealable plastic bags in the freezer. The rules for what to save and what should be in the garbage disposal involve common sense. You can use wilted vegetables, as long as they are not obviously rotten, dirty, or contaminated. Wash all vegetables before peeling or slicing. Keep the "sweet" vegetables in equal or higher proportion to "strong tasting" vegetables. For example, carrots, celery, apple cores and peelings, sweet peppers, winter squash, and onions will give your broth a gentle sweetness. On the other hand, too much cabbage, broccoli, or strong greens will give your broth an unpleasant overtone. Chicken broth has a delicate flavor, and, for that reason, you will want fewer strong veggies. Wait until you see chicken on sale and then buy in quantity, freezing it for future use if you're not ready to make broth immediately.

If you do this right, your broth will be more concentrated than the watery conventional brands, so you may need to adjust your own recipes accordingly. June

Prep Time: 1 to 2 hours (including straining at the end)
Cook Time: 3 hours or longer

Ingredients:

6 quarts of liquid from list below
Approximately 10 lbs. whole chickens, parts, chicken thighs, etc.
2 to 3 1-gallon freezer bags of saved vegetable scraps
4 bay leaves

Kitchen Tools:

Large stockpot
Large strainer
Splatter screen
Large bowl or stockpot to drain broth into
Several freezer containers in sizes that makes sense for you
Potato masher

Instructions:

1. Thaw any liquids you have been saving and heat in stockpot.
2. Thaw chicken and wash in cold water to reduce bacteria. Cut up chicken if you are using whole birds. Thaw vegetable scraps in the microwave and add to the stockpot along with the bay leaves. Liquid should almost cover the chicken and vegetables, as additional juices will be naturally generated upon cooking. **Do not add salt.**
3. Turn stove on high until mixture boils, cover, and reduce heat to low. Simmer for a minimum of 3 hours and up to 5 hours. There's no exact science here—just make sure the liquid doesn't boil away. Remove from heat and let cool a bit.
4. Place a sturdy strainer over a large, deep bowl or pan. Ladle cooked vegetables, meat and liquid into the strainer a few cups at a time. Press down to squeeze out juices (a potato masher works great here), and when well drained, dispose of the pulp. Repeat the process until the entire batch has been strained.
5. Wash out the original stockpot or use another large pot or bowl. Using a splatter screen, strain the liquid a second time to eliminate seeds and any small particles. If your freezer space is at a premium, return the broth to the stove and continue to cook until broth is reduced by half. This intensifies the flavor and, upon use, simply use 1 part broth with 1 part water.
6. Cool broth in the freezer long enough for the fat to form a solid layer on the top and remove the fat. Or if you are out of time and/or patience, simply pour broth into freezer containers and freeze. Fat will rise to the top. To easily remove fat, microwave frozen broth on high for 1 to 2 minutes and "peel" off fat.
7. Label each container with not only what it is, but also the date to make it easier to rotate broth. Also note on the label whether you've reduced the broth so it is extra rich. Use in soups, gravies, casseroles, and in place of water in most savory recipes.

See Beef Broth for Usable Ingredients, Liquids to Use, Ingredients to Limit, and What <u>Not</u> to Include

Vegetable Broth

When we determined to read every label on every packaged food, we didn't think finding a vegetable broth without sugar, yeast, tomato, or MSG would be an issue. We were so wrong. We prefer to use broth instead of water in most recipes and the alternative to the packaged broths was to cook up our own. I have used this formula for 30 years, and my kids teasingly called it "Garbage Soup." I never took offense because there were never any complaints when it was used in soups and other dishes.

We save all our vegetable scraps and peelings in gallon sized resealable plastic bags in the freezer. The rules for what to save and what should be in the garbage disposal involve common sense. You can use wilted vegetables, as long as they are not obviously rotten, dirty, or contaminated. Wash all vegetables before peeling or slicing. Keep the "sweet" vegetables in equal or higher proportion to "strong tasting" vegetables. For example, carrots, celery, apple cores and peelings, sweet peppers, winter squash, and onions will give your broth a gentle sweetness. On the other hand, too much cabbage, broccoli, or strong greens will give your broth an unpleasant overtone. You'll get it figured out as you go along, and, although it takes some time to do this, you'll be so much healthier, and your dishes will taste better. June

Prep Time: 1 to 2 hours (including straining at the end)
Cook Time: 2 to 4 hours

Ingredients:

6 quarts of liquid from list below
3 to 4 1-gallon freezer bags of saved vegetable scraps
4 bay leaves

Kitchen Tools:

Large stockpot
Large strainer
Splatter screen
Large bowl or stockpot to drain broth into
Several freezer containers in sizes that makes sense for you
Potato masher

Instructions:

1. Thaw any liquids you have been saving and heat in stockpot.
2. Thaw vegetable scraps in the microwave and add to the stockpot. You should be able to see the liquid when you press down on vegetables but not cover the vegetables, as additional juices will be naturally generated upon cooking. **Do not add salt.**
3. Turn stove on high until mixture boils, cover, and reduce heat to low. Simmer for no less than 2 hours but preferably up to 4 hours, stirring occasionally. There's no exact science here—make sure the liquid doesn't boil away and vegetables don't burn onto bottom of the pan. Remove from heat and let cool a bit.
4. Using a sturdy strainer over a large, deep bowl or pan, ladle cooked vegetables and liquid into the strainer a few cups at a time. Press down to squeeze out juices (a potato masher works great here), and when well drained, dispose of the pulp. Repeat the process until the entire batch has been strained.
5. Wash out the original stockpot or use another large pot or bowl. Using a splatter screen, strain the liquid a second time to eliminate seeds and any small particles. If your freezer space is at a premium, return the broth to the stove and continue to cook until broth is reduced by half. This intensifies the flavor and, upon use, simply use 1 part broth with 1 part water.
6. Label each container, with not only what it is, but also the date to make it easier to rotate broth. Also note on the label whether you've reduced the broth so it is extra rich. Use in soups, gravies, casseroles, and in place of water in most savory recipes.

See Beef Broth for Usable Ingredients, Liquids to Use, Ingredients to Limit, and What Not to Include

Bette Hagman's Modified GF Flour Mix

We are deeply grateful to Bette Hagman for her many years of research and recipe development. In the mid-1970s, when she was diagnosed with Celiac Disease, there was little information available. She put her energies into developing recipes for foods she liked, and eventually published them to help others on this same gluten-free journey. Her series of cookbooks, The Gluten-Free Gourmet, published by Henry Holt and Company, offer a tremendous variety of delicious, gluten-free dishes.

Bette's original recipe for gluten-free flour calls for arrowroot starch, and we have swapped out cornstarch just because of cost. We found the substitution made no difference in our recipes. This flour mix can generally be exchanged cup for cup with wheat flour, and we use it when a recipe calls for a nonspecific gluten free flour mix. We offer it here with our sincere thanks to Ms. Hagman for being a pioneer in the industry, and her tireless focus on making the difficult transition to a gluten-free diet a little easier. June

Prep Time: 5 minutes

Ingredients:

For 6 cups	**For 3 cups**
4 cups white rice flour	2 cups white rice flour
1 1/3 cups potato starch	2/3 cup potato starch
2/3 cup cornstarch	1/3 cup cornstarch

Kitchen Tools:

Measuring cups

Bowl to mix

Convenient container to store flour

Instructions:

1. Measure out ingredients and mix thoroughly. Store in an airtight, labeled container. This flour mix does not require refrigeration.

Bette Hagman's Featherlight Flour Mix

We have a special appreciation for Bette Hagman's amazing cookbook, The Gluten-free Gourmet Cooks Comfort Foods, copyright 2004, published by Henry Holt and Company. It was one of the first cookbooks we found that had wonderful, sensible recipes that tasted like the foods we had grown up with. After discovering Kris was Celiac and Jonathan was gluten intolerant, we needed more normalcy in our lives. Bette Hagman's cookbook series made us excited about cooking and baking again.

We were introduced to Ms. Hagman's Featherlight Flour Mix through many of her recipes, and the light consistency of baked goods were beyond our expectations of gluten-free flours. We offer it here with our sincere thanks to Ms. Hagman. June

Prep Time: 5 minutes

Ingredients:

For 6 cups

2 cups rice flour

2 cups tapioca flour

2 cups cornstarch

2 tablespoons potato flour
(not potato starch)

For 3 cups

1 cup rice flour

1 cup tapioca flour

1 cup cornstarch

1 tablespoon potato flour

Kitchen Tools:

Measuring cup and spoon

Bowl to mix

Convenient container to store flour

Instructions:

1. Measure out ingredients and mix thoroughly. Store in an airtight, labeled container. This flour mix does not require refrigeration.

Five Flour Mix

Bean flour adds a tenderness and color to baked goods, that rice flour won't accomplish on its own. Most bean flour mixes call for sorghum flour, also known as jowar or milo. Unfortunately, Kris is allergic to sorghum, and it was necessary to find a substitute. We found a combination of brown rice flour and corn flour make a viable alternative to sorghum in baked goods.

There are many bean flours, some of which can be found in oriental markets. They go by different names—garbanzo, garfava, gram, chickpea, or besan, plus a few more combination flours under separate names we probably aren't aware of. We use gram and besan because of availability and low cost. They tend to clump together, so to avoid sifting, simply put the flour in your blender for a bit or use a whisk and a gentle hand. June

Makes: 9 cups
Prep Time: 5 minutes

Ingredients:

3 cups cornstarch
3 cups tapioca flour
2 cups bean flour (garfava, besan, gram, chickpea, garbanzo or combination)
1/2 cup corn flour (not masa harina)
1/2 cup brown rice flour

Kitchen Tools:

Large bowl
Stirring spoon
Measuring cups

Instructions:

1. Thoroughly but gently stir to combine all ingredients in a large bowl, and store in an airtight, labeled container. This flour mix does not require refrigeration.

Celery Salt

Celery salt has only two ingredients, but you may need to purchase ground celery seed from an internet store. In our area of the east coast, ground celery seed is not available in brick and mortar stores. Check out www.myspicesage.com for a huge selection of herbs and spices.

Perhaps you have never used celery salt. If not, experiment combining it with eggs, vegetables, or a tossed salad with simply fresh lemon juice and oil as a dressing. June

Prep Time: 3 minutes

Ingredients:

2 parts sea salt

1 part ground celery seed

Kitchen Tools:

Measuring spoon

Small bowl

Storage container

Instructions:

1. Combine salt and celery seed in a small bowl and mix well. Pour into a labeled storage container.

Dill Seasoning

This seasoning mixture was invented when I needed a combination that would accentuate the subtle flavor of cucumber. The dill, onion, and garlic meld together, and work well with many other gentle flavors, such as eggs. Experiment with it and see what foods you can enhance. June

Prep Time: 5 minutes

Ingredients:

4 parts dried dill weed

2 parts onion powder

1 part garlic powder

Kitchen Tools:

Measuring spoons

Small bowl

Storage container

Instructions:

1. Combine all ingredients in a small bowl and mix well. Pour into a labeled storage container.

Ginger-Free Pumpkin Pie Spice

If you have an allergy to ginger or simply don't like it, you may have discovered that ginger is one of the traditional ingredients in pumpkin pie spice. It's easy to work around this ingredient by using a combination of four pungent spices that love each other.

While the ingredients for this mix are simple and few, the taste is stunning. Be sure to keep it in a dry, dark cupboard in a closed container. June

Prep Time: 3 minutes

Ingredients:

1 tablespoon ground cinnamon

1 1/2 teaspoons ground allspice

1 teaspoon ground nutmeg

1/2 teaspoon ground cloves

Kitchen Tools:

Measuring spoons

Small bowl

Storage container

Instructions:

1. Combine all ingredients in a small bowl and mix well. Pour into a labeled storage container.

Italian Herb Mix

Italian seasoning is quite expensive in the store, yet reasonably inexpensive to make. If you Google recipes, you will see a wide range of possibilities. We particularly like this combination of herbs. Add it to green beans, your favorite soups, or get creative.

Dried herbs have a shelf life so be sure to keep all your herbs in a dark cupboard, away from your stove, preferably at 70 degrees or cooler. Under those conditions, your herbs should last a year. June

Prep Time: 5 minutes

Ingredients:

2 parts dried basil

2 parts dried oregano

1 part dried rosemary

1 part dried savory

1 part rubbed sage

1 part dried marjoram

Kitchen Tools:

Measuring spoons

Small bowl

Storage container

Instructions:

1. Combine all ingredients in a small bowl and mix well. Pour into a labeled storage container.

Thymeless Mediterranean Herb Mix

When Kris realized thyme did not agree with her or her digestive tract, we had to rethink and reread the labels on our purchased herb mixes. Just as we suspected, almost all of them contained some quantity of thyme. The alternative was to put together our own thymeless herb mix. After some research and experimentation, we found the bold flavor of savory to be a suitable substitution for thyme.

We particularly like this mixture in beef dishes. June

Prep Time: 5 minutes

Ingredients:

3 tablespoons parsley flakes

3 tablespoons chopped dried onion

1 tablespoon plus 1 1/2 teaspoons dried basil

1 tablespoon plus 1 1/2 teaspoons grated lemon peel, dried

1 teaspoon ground celery seed

1 teaspoon ground savory

1 teaspoon ground marjoram

Kitchen Tools:

Measuring spoons

Small bowl

Storage container

Mini food processor

Instructions:

1. Place chopped, dried onion in a mini food processor and pulse briefly to break up into smaller bits, being careful not to make it into onion powder. An alternative method is to use a mortar and pestle.
2. Combine all ingredients in a small bowl and mix well. Pour into a labeled storage container.

Seasoned Salt

Sister Mary Butzer, one of my dearest friends for over 40 years, graciously shared this family recipe with me. Her mother, Frances Rock Butzer was born in 1904. The devoted wife of a physician who made house calls, she was brilliant in her own right and raised 12 children in Mankato, Minnesota. Upon her death, and in the process of cleaning out her house, the daughters found all the spices and herbs needed to make the seasoned salt, but the recipe had been lost over the years. It was later found, in Mrs. Butzer's precious handwriting, and once again redistributed to the family. I'm honored to include it here with some modifications. June

Makes: 4 cups
Prep Time: 5 minutes

Ingredients:

3 cups course salt
1/4 cup ground celery seed
1/4 cup onion powder
1/4 cup garlic powder
1/4 cup paprika
2 tablespoons nutmeg

Kitchen Tools:

Large bowl
Spoon or whisk for mixing
Glass jars for storage

Instructions:

1. Pour all ingredients into a bowl and mix well.
2. Store in labeled glass jars to keep it dry. It will keep for years, but guaranteed not to last that long. We love sharing samples with friends!

Original Recipe: The original recipe called for celery salt, onion salt, garlic salt, and 2 tablespoons of sugar. I've used ground celery seed, onion powder, and garlic powder to enhance the flavor and cut down on the salt content. I also eliminated the sugar.

Taco Seasoning

Tacos are one of Kris's favorite foods, but each time we made them, she got sick. After reading the label on every taco mix in the store (which took about 1 minute because the choices were slim), we discovered why—they contained milk solids and sugar, both triggers for Candida. It didn't take long for me to locate several recipes for taco mixes in cookbooks and the internet.

There really are no mysterious, exotic ingredients needed to make great tacos. You might already have what you need in your cupboard. Taco seasoning is easy to make, healthier, and costs far less than the packaged kind. We particularly like this combination, but make it your own by adding or subtracting to suit your taste. June

Makes: Approximately 4 oz. or enough for 8 lbs. ground beef
Prep Time: 10 minutes

Ingredients:

4 tablespoons chili powder
3 tablespoons cumin
3 tablespoons paprika
2 tablespoons onion powder
2 tablespoons garlic powder
1 tablespoon potato starch
1 teaspoon Seasoned Salt (see recipe in this section)
1/4 to 1/2 teaspoon cayenne pepper

Kitchen Tools:

Jar or container with a tight lid
Measuring spoons

Instructions:

1. Combine all ingredients in a labeled jar and shake to combine. Store in your cupboard out of direct sunlight.
2. Use 2 tablespoons of mix or more per pound of hamburger.

Onion Soup & Dip Mix

Early in our gluten-free journey, we were thrilled to find a dry onion soup and dip mix online. The taste was reminiscent of the old fashioned dry Lipton Onion Soup that came in packets, and could spice up a meat loaf, become the base of a soup, or be mixed with almost any savory ingredient. This online version was certified organic, gluten free, tasty, and, for a while, it was a winner.

Periodically, we sweep through our cupboards to reread all the labels, just to make sure something hasn't slipped past us, or to look for an ingredient that Kris is now allergic to. Much to our dismay, we discovered the dry soup mix contained maltodextrin, which has become an extremely common ingredient in processed foods.

Maltodextrin is a sugar derived from any number of foods—corn, barley, wheat, rice, or potato starch to name a few. Maltodextrin is so highly processed, that it is considered gluten free, but being a sugar, it can feed Candida. We avoid all sugars as much as possible.

This recipe for Onion Soup & Dip Mix is easy to make, inexpensive, and has none of the harmful ingredients in branded mixes. Get creative with it: use it in gravies, meat loaf, casseroles, or any food that needs a bit of flavor. June

Makes: Approximately 1 3/4 cups

Prep Time: 10 minutes

Ingredients:

1 cup chopped dried onion
1/4 cup onion powder
1/4 cup potato flour
3 tablespoons sea salt
2 tablespoons garlic powder
1 teaspoon ground celery seed
1 teaspoon ground pepper

Kitchen Tools:

Jar or container with a tight lid
Measuring cups and spoons

Instructions:

1. If dried onion is of coarse consistency, put it in a food processor and carefully pulse until pieces are 1/4" or a little smaller. Too much pulsing will turn it into onion powder. Pour into a bowl.
2. Add all other ingredients and stir to combine. Store in a labeled container in your cupboard out of direct sunlight. Stir before using.
3. Experiment with various quantities mixed with meats, vegetables, or rice dishes.

How To

We turn to this How To section a lot, and think you will too. It does not contain recipes, but gives you formulas and techniques for doing things to get optimum results. Each one is essential to know, and we offer it as a quick guide for your convenience.

How to Cook Quinoa stresses the need to wash the bitter coating off this versatile grain before cooking, and explains how to attain a perfectly unfurled grain. How to Hard Boil Eggs will keep you from having green yolks. Use this section as a handy reference for how long and at what temperatures to bake squashes. Be sure to check out How to Season Wood. Any wooden utensil and cutting board you have will love this treatment.

So, browse through this section and come back to it when you need it.

How to Cook Rice

The texture and taste of rice makes it a versatile side dish, or part of a main course. Long grain brown or white rice will give you rice that separates after cooking. Short grain rice comes in either brown or white, and will give you a sticky rice when cooked. There are vast varieties of rice, some of which are domestic, and a lot of wonderful imported varieties. Try black, red, or purple rice, which can be found in health food stores or in almost every international market.

Most rice is coated with something to keep the kernels from sticking together, and can be rice powder, powdered glucose, or talc. Unless stated otherwise on the packaging, all rice must be washed in cold water to remove the coating before cooking. June

Makes: Approximately 3 cups
Prep Time: 5 minutes
Cook Time: 30 minutes

Ingredients:

1 cup uncooked brown or white long grain rice
1 3/4 cups water
1 teaspoon salt

Kitchen Tools:

2-quart saucepan
Measuring cups

Instructions:

1. Measure rice and put in the saucepan. Fill with enough cold water to gently swish the rice around with your hands. Drain off water, and repeat the process two more times to remove the outer coating.
2. Add 1 3/4 cups cold water, salts and heat to boiling. Reduce heat to low, cover, and simmer 30 minutes or until all moisture is absorbed. Do not lift the lid, as the steam helps cook the rice. Remove from heat and fluff rice with a fork.

How to Cook Quinoa

Quinoa (pronounced KEEN' wah) is an ancient grain that dates back at least 5000 years to the Aztecs, and is still a staple food for the South American Indians living in the Andes Mountains. Quinoa is able to grow in high altitudes and withstand frost and intense sun. It was first imported to the United States in the 1970s, and has grown in popularity due to its superior nutritional qualities and versatility. Quinoa is considered a complete protein, as it includes all nine essential amino acids.

If you read the quinoa packaging, you will see a ratio of 1:2 for quinoa to liquid, which produces cooked quinoa that clumps together. Using less liquid will give you a light, fluffy quinoa, and this is the method we prefer. Quinoa continues to expand in liquids, so plan your dishes accordingly. June

Makes: 4 cups
Prep Time: 5 minutes
Cook Time: 15 to 20 minutes

Ingredients:

1 cup quinoa

1 1/4 cups water

Kitchen Tools:

2-quart saucepan

Measuring cups

Splatter screen

Instructions:

1. Measure quinoa and put in the saucepan. Fill with enough cold water to gently wash the quinoa. Using a splatter screen held firmly over the top of the pan, pour off the water. Repeat the process at least two more times.
2. Add 1 1/4 cups cold water and heat to boiling. Reduce heat to low, cover, and simmer for 15 to 20 minutes or until all moisture is absorbed. Remove from heat and let rest, still covered, for another 5 minutes. Fluff and serve instead of rice, in soups, stews, or salads.

How to Cook Spaghetti Squash

Spaghetti squash is a seasonal vegetable, harvested in the fall, and available through fall, winter, and early spring in grocery stores. An uncut squash will keep for up to a month in a cool dry place. When choosing squash, look for a creamy yellow shell, free of soft or dark spots. While squash can be microwaved or boiled, we like the flavor of baked squash. When properly cooked, the squash will produce spaghetti-like strands that can be removed with a fork. Serve this low-calorie vegetable hot with buttery spread, salt and pepper, or in place of pasta. Kris

Serves: 4
Prep Time: 5 minutes
Bake Time: 30 to 40 minutes

Ingredients:

1 spaghetti squash
Oil for pan

Kitchen Tools:

Baking pan
Secure cutting board
Sharp long-bladed knife
Spoon (to scoop out seeds)

Instructions:

1. Preheat oven to 375 degrees F (191 degrees C). Oil baking pan and set aside.
2. Wash the squash shell with soap and water, rinsing well, so bacteria is not dragged through the squash as it's cut. Squash should be cut in half the long way. Placing it on a secure cutting board and holding it firmly, place the tip of your knife into the center of the squash and use the leverage of the handle to cut through the squash. Turn it around and cut through the other side. Your goal is to cut it so both halves are equal.
3. Using a tablespoon, scoop out the stringy center holding the seeds, and discard or reserve for making broth. Place cut side down in baking dish, and bake for 30 to 40 minutes, until squash easily fluffs out in strings. A pronged spaghetti server works great for this purpose. If baked too long, it will turn to mush.
4. Serve hot with buttery spread and your favorite seasonings, or as a base for any dish in which you would use spaghetti.

How To Cook Winter Squash

Winter squash comes in many different sizes, shapes, colors, and varieties, and the best part is that there are always at least two varieties or more available all year around. You'll most often see acorn and butternut squash, but do some research and check out your local oriental market for new delights. Each type has its own particular taste, and you probably already have your favorites. Some squash lends itself well to peeling and boiling, but we prefer to keep the flavor intact throughout baking. This method is simple and, best of all, once it goes in the oven, you can set the timer and forget about it. This is simply a basic guide to launch your creativity for a versatile vegetable. Kris

Serves: 4
Prep Time: 5 minutes
Bake Time: 40 to 60 minutes depending on size

Ingredients:
1 winter squash
Oil for pan

Kitchen Tools:
Baking pan
Secure cutting board
Sharp long-bladed knife
Spoon (to scoop out seeds)

Instructions:

1. Preheat oven to 375 degrees F (191 degrees C). Oil baking pan and set aside.
2. Wash the squash shell with soap and water, rinsing well so bacteria is not dragged through the squash as it's cut. Squash should be cut in half the long way for oval varieties. Placing it on a secure cutting board, and holding it firmly, place the tip of your knife into the center of squash and use the leverage of the handle to cut through the squash. Turn it around and cut through the other side. Your goal is to cut it so both halves are equal.
3. Using a tablespoon, scoop out the stringy center including seeds, and discard or reserve for making broth. Place cut side down in baking dish, and bake for 40 to 60 minutes, until a fork will easily push into the center or the thickest part of the squash.
4. Serve hot with buttery spread and your favorite seasonings.

How To Hard Boil Eggs

While it sounds like something out a Dr. Seuss book, you, like me, have probably ended up with green eggs at one time or another, which is what happens to the yolks if the eggs are boiled too long. The colorful yolks are caused by iron in the yolks that reacts with hydrogen sulfide from the whites, according to the American Egg Board. While the discoloration is harmless, we have included a foolproof recipe for hard boiling eggs, just in case green isn't your favorite color.

You have probably found it as frustrating as we have when hard boiled eggs do not peel easily. Fifty years ago, as a young bride, I bought eggs from a farmer in rural North Dakota. The farmer asked if I was going to hard boil them or use them in baking. When I asked what difference that could possibly make, she told me fresh laid eggs do not peel easily. Her explanation sounded so fanciful as it ricocheted off the corners of my brain, that I didn't have the sense to ask why or how it could be true. I also regret not asking how old eggs had to be to peel easily. Best guess is to ensure your eggs sit in your fridge for a week before boiling.

When peeling, rap egg against a hard surface until all sides are cracked. Then gently roll the egg under the palm of your hand for a bit and, if all else fails, try peeling under cold running water. June

Cook Time: 15 to 18 minutes
Cooling Time: 10 to 20 minutes

Kitchen Tools:
Pan with tight fitting lid

Instructions:

1. Gently place eggs in a saucepan and completely cover with cold water.
2. Turn heat on high and watch eggs carefully until the water comes to a full boil.
3. Cover pan, shut off heat, and set timer for 15 to 18 minutes.
4. When timer goes off, immediately pour off hot water, and fill pan with cold water. In a minute or so, pour off the now warm water, fill pan again with cold water, and allow eggs to cool. When sufficiently cooled, store eggs in the refrigerator.

How To Roast A Whole Chicken

In times past, we would pick up a whole, already roasted chicken from the grocery store for a quick, tasty meal. The crisp skin and seasonings were delicious, but often had ingredients we'd rather not eat or simply could not have. At times like that, we always turned to Betty Crocker's New Picture Cookbook, published by McGraw Hill Book Company, circa 1961.

We learned that roasting a whole chicken is easy and allows you to vary your seasonings to your own taste. For a simple but satisfying taste, sprinkle with seasoned salt and roast. For an Italian flair, season with salt and pepper along with Italian seasoning. You are limited only by your taste buds and imagination. Kris

Roast Time: 1 hour 30 minutes to 2 hours depending on weight

Kitchen Tools:

Roasting pan

Instructions:

1. If chicken is frozen, allow enough time for it to thaw in a safe way—in the refrigerator or in cold water. Safely defrosting does not include microwaving!
2. Preheat oven to 375 degrees F (191 degrees C). Oil a shallow baking dish large enough to hold the chicken with a little extra room.
3. Wash the chicken under cold running water, using your fingers to ensure all areas of skin folds are rinsed off. Remove any residual internal organs from the inside and rinse well. Pat dry with paper towels.
4. Either spray or rub oil of your choice on all sides of the chicken, and place in pan with **breast side down**. Sprinkle your favorite seasonings as evenly as possible over the chicken. Turn chicken over and repeat the process.
5. Bake uncovered, **breast side up** using the following formula, depending on weight of the chicken:
   - 4 to 5 lbs. bake for 1 hour 30 minutes to 1 hour 45 minutes
   - Over 5 lbs. bake for 1 hour 45 minutes to 2 hours
6. Baste juices over chicken occasionally as it bakes.

How To Store Lettuce

Most lettuce grows in heads, either tightly compacted or loose heads. Other lettuce grows as leaves on a stem. Each type has its own particular shape, color, and taste, so experiment to determine what works best for you and your palate. Here's a rundown of the most common lettuces on the market:

Most commonly known is ***iceberg lettuce****, with crisp very pale leaves and little taste. It has almost no nutritional value and is best combined with other greens to make the most of its texture.*

Boston *or* ***Bibb lettuce*** *is pale green with round, delicate leaves in loosely packed heads. The taste is gentle and sweet.*

Green leaf *and* ***red leaf lettuce*** *grow in loose heads with delicate ruffled edges. The taste is mild and leaves must be treated gently when washing.*

Romaine *grows in large, elongated heads and is exceptionally crisp, which is why it's used in Caesar salad. The leaves are large enough to wrap around meats and vegetables for a change from wrap breads.*

Arugula *grows on stems, not heads, and has a slightly peppery taste. The broad, flat leaves are best mixed with other types of lettuce.*

Radicchio *has a bitter taste and is unmistakable with its burgundy colored, tightly compacted leaves streaked with white stems.*

Watercress *is grown in water with small leaves on delicate, hollow stems. It has a slightly peppery taste and works well in Asian soups.*

Oak leaf lettuce *gets its name from its resemblance to oak leaves and is a delicate green in color. It's most often seen in lettuce mixes, and has a mild, sweet taste similar to Boston lettuce.*

Curly endive *grows in a small head and has very thin, ruffled leaves on each stem. It is most often seen in packaged lettuce mixes, and the taste is a bit bitter.*

Belgian endive *has a bitter taste and grows in compact, elongated heads with pale green leaves at the top and white stems. It is best combined with mild lettuces.*

Escarole *grows in a head with broad, slightly bitter, ruffled leaves. Outer leaves are most often used in soups and stews, while the inner leaves are more appropriate for salads.*

With all the varieties of lettuce offering a vast array of textures and taste available in almost every standard grocery store, there's no excuse for having a boring salad. Experiment and enjoy the variety of greens available. June

Instructions:

1. Choose lettuce that is crisp and healthy looking. Remove the leaves from the stalks, and gently wash in cool but not ice cold water. Transfer to a strainer. Check the bottom of the pan, and if there is any grit, pour off the water and repeat the process as many times as necessary until there is no more grit in the bottom of the pan.
2. To store, use a clean, cotton dishtowel (not the terry cloth type) and lay it out on a flat surface. Place clean lettuce in single layer on a small portion of the towel. Gently fold an edge of the towel over the lettuce and repeat the process, having a layer of towel between the layers of lettuce. Any lettuce leaves that overlap each other will deteriorate first. Store in a plastic bag in your vegetable crisper for up to two weeks.

How To Prepare & Store Fresh Parsley

There is just nothing like the scent and taste of fresh parsley, and if you've never used it, you're in for a treat! Some of our recipes call for fresh parsley and, in all cases, it's just not the same if you try to substitute dried parsley. Most stores carry at least one kind of parsley, and often two.

Italian parsley has a flat, lobed leaf, and is preferred by chefs because it is easier to work with, and dirt is less apt to get caught in the leaves. Don't confuse it with cilantro, which has a similar leaf but tastes totally different. They are not interchangeable.

Curly leaf parsley is the traditional parsley you see as a garnish on your plate in restaurants. It is as flavorful as flat leaf parsley, but requires a little more attention in the washing process to remove any grit from its leaves.

Parsley must be carefully washed and, if stored properly, will keep for two weeks in your refrigerator. Here's the process. June

Instructions:

1. Choose parsley that is dark green and crisp. Bypass any that is limp, as it hasn't been displayed properly in the store. If you are not going to use it immediately, put it in a plastic bag in your vegetable crisper for no more than a few days.
2. Unwrap the parsley bunch and plunge it in a sufficient amount of cool but not ice cold water to wash it. Ice water will wilt the parsley. Discard any light green or brown wilted sprigs.
3. Taking each stem, one by one, give it a gentle swish in the water and pinch off each clump of leaves from the stem. If you save your vegetable scraps for making your own broth, set the stems aside for this purpose, and put the leaves in a bowl or strainer. Continue this process until you have separated all the leaves from the stems.
4. If there is any grit in the bottom of the pan, rinse out the pan, fill it with cool water, and wash the parsley leaves again. Continue to follow this process until there is no more dirt in the bottom of the pan, and then wash the parsley one more time just to be sure. Any grit left in the parsley will ruin your dish!
5. Remove parsley from the water and shake out excess water.
6. To store your clean parsley, place a paper towel in the bottom of a large bowl. Put a single layer of parsley leaves on the paper towel and fold the corners of the paper towel inward to make a dry layer. Put a single layer of parsley on the paper towel, and place another paper towel on top. Continue to layer the parsley between dry paper towels, ending with a paper towel.
7. Cover the bowl and refrigerate for up to 2 weeks.

How To Season Wooden Utensils

Raw wood needs to be treated or cured before use to prevent bacteria growth, and to enable wooden utensils to repel liquids. An extremely knowledgeable mountain-climbing friend of mine in the wood business shared this formula with me. I was unable to verify the origins of the formula, but I can attest that the process works.

Peanut oil is generally recommended, but since peanut allergies are on the rise, we recommend mineral oil, a non-toxic substitute you can purchase at most hardware stores or pharmacies.

It's best to resist the urge to put wooden utensils in your dishwasher. Hand washing is recommended to preserve the seasoning.

If you follow the prescribed formula below, you'll have many years of use from your cutting boards and wooden utensils. To ensure you complete the treatment as prescribed, we recommend you mark on your calendar each date of treatment required. If cared for properly, your boards and wooden utensils will last a lifetime and can even be passed on to your children. June

Instructions:

1. Apply mineral oil liberally to all surfaces and edges, every day for a week. Allow oil to soak in and wipe off excess oil at the end of the week. You may begin using your wooden utensils at this point, as long as you continue the seasoning process.
2. Treat wood once a week for 2 months. Let oil soak into wood for a couple hours and then wipe off excess.
3. Treat wood once a month for 6 months. Let oil soak into wood for a couple hours and then wipe off excess.
4. Treat wood once a year every year after that. Let oil soak into wood for a couple hours and then wipe off excess.

Index

A

B

C

Coconut

D

Daiya

E

F

G

H

I

J

K

L

M

N

O

P

Q

R

S

T

V

W

X

Y

Z

Made in the USA
Middletown, DE
09 October 2025

18988199R00234